Promoting Social Interaction for Individuals with Communicative Impairments

of related interest

From Isolation to Intimacy
Making Friends without Words
Phoebe Caldwell with Jane Horwood
ISBN 978 1 84310 500 8

Finding You Finding Me
Using Intensive Interaction to Get in Touch with People whose Severe
Learning Disabilities are Combined with Autistic Spectrum Disorder
Phoebe Caldwell
ISBN 978 1 84310 399 8

Communication Issues in Autism and Asperger Syndrome
Do we speak the same language?
Olga Bogdashina
ISBN 978 1 84310 267 0

Assessing and Developing Communication and Thinking Skills
in People with Autism and Communication Difficulties
A Toolkit for Parents and Professionals
Kate Silver with Autism Initiatives
ISBN 978 1 84310 352 3

Music Therapy, Sensory Integration and the Autistic Child
Dorita S. Berger
Foreword by Donna Williams
ISBN 978 1 84310 700 2

I Dreamed I was Normal
A Music Therapist's Journey into the Realms of Autism
Ginger Clarkson
ISBN 978 1 58106 007 2

Getting IT
Using Information Technology to Empower People with Communication
Difficulties
Dinah Murray and Ann Aspinall
ISBN 978 1 84310 375 2

Understanding Learning Disability and Dementia
Developing Effective Interventions
Diana Kerr
ISBN 978 1 84310 442 1

Promoting Social Interaction for Individuals with Communicative Impairments

Making Contact

Edited by M. Suzanne Zeedyk

Jessica Kingsley Publishers
London and Philadelphia

First published in 2008
by Jessica Kingsley Publishers
116 Pentonville Road
London N1 9JB, UK
and
400 Market Street, Suite 400
Philadelphia, PA 19106, USA

www.jkp.com

Library of Congress Cataloging in Publication Data
Promoting social interaction for individuals with communicative impairments : making contact / edited by M. Suzanne Zeedyk.
    p. cm.
    ISBN 978-1-84310-539-8 (pb : alk. paper) 1. People with disabilities--Means of communication. 2. Communicative disorders--Patients--Rehabilitation. 3. Communicative disorders--Social aspects. I. Zeedyk, M. Suzanne (Mary Suzanne), 1963-
    HV1568.4.M35 2008
    362.4'048--dc22

                                2007042992

British Library Cataloguing in Publication Data
A CIP catalogue record for this book is available from the British Library

ISBN 978 1 84310 539 8

Printed and bound in Great Britain by
Athenaeum Press, Gateshead, Tyne and Wear

Contents

Part 3: A Closer Look at Interventions

CHAPTER I

INTRODUCTION: BRIDGING A SPECTRUM OF COMMUNICATIVE IMPAIRMENTS

M. Suzanne Zeedyk

We humans are social creatures. We need to engage with other people, to laugh with them, share stories with them, negotiate plans with them and sit comfortably in silence with them. There is growing interest, across a wide range of scientific and societal domains, in this process of human communication. Parents are urged to spend more time talking to their pre-verbal babies (e.g. National Literacy Trust 2007). Television programmes are made highlighting the long hours that elderly people spend isolated in the rooms of their care homes (e.g. Rage Against the Darkness 2004). Computer games are developed as a means of teaching autistic children the skills of making conversation with peers (e.g. Parsons and Mitchell 2002). Waiters are advised that they can earn more tips by speaking to customers in a certain manner (e.g. Van Baaren 2005). What a broad and disparate range of concerns!

The aim of this book is to counter that impression of diversity. Such issues are not disconnected and separate. They have an underlying base that gives them more commonalities than may at first be apparent. Recognising this unity across domains can foster both theoretical and applied insights. For example, understanding that infants are born already able to communicate with other people can help in designing more effective interventions for children with autism. Knowing that deafblind people have the (often unrecognised) capacity for complex conversational exchanges provides clues about the emergence of language in human evolutionary history. Reflecting on the ways in which we all sometimes feel anxious and short-tempered enables us to reinterpret aggressive behaviour in adults with learning disabilities as distress, rather than as violence. Such domains would normally be explored singularly, in books that focus on a specific domain. Our purpose in this volume is to take the opposite approach, bringing together a set of apparently diverse concerns within the same volume. We have two complementary goals in mind in doing so, the first being to share with a wider audience some of the scientific insights that interdisciplinary approaches to the field of human communication are yielding. The second is to illustrate how those insights are being used to develop novel interventions for communicative abilities that have become impaired.

The contributors to this volume come from a range of backgrounds. Some are practitioners who work regularly with clients with some form of communicative challenge. Their chapters offer wisdom gained from their practical experience. Other contributors are researchers, who describe the empirical studies that they have been conducting. Some of the work they discuss focuses on basic processes of human communication, while other efforts aim to systematically evaluate the effectiveness of intervention techniques. It is still somewhat unusual to bring together researchers and practitioners, because their terminologies and their concerns can differ remarkably, but we hope that the contents of this volume demonstrate the benefits that exist for both readers and contributors in crossing over traditional boundaries.

One might wonder how this mixed group came to be working together. The immediate background to the volume was a public seminar held in Dundee, Scotland, in 2007, entitled 'Promoting Social Interaction for Individuals with Profound Communication Needs', at which all of the authors presented their work to an audience of 150 people interested in the area of communication. The interest was more extensive than anticipated, with special needs teachers, mental health nurses, speech and language therapists, occupational therapists, care staff, parents, academics, students, and even musicians and artists attending. Feedback indicated that the most compelling aspects of the event for the delegates were links that they discovered with domains that they had previously had little familiarity with. For example, the challenges some faced in working with, say, children who had suffered severe neglect began to take on new meaning when it became apparent that similar challenges were being faced by staff working with elderly people with dementia. Many delegates also expressed frustration that the time constraints of the day meant that they could attend only a few of the workshops on offer. Thus this book was born, out of a sense that it would make the full content of the seminar available to all who were interested – not only those who attended on the day, but also an extended, international audience. This also meant that the investment made by the Developmental Section of the British Psychological Society, who kindly provided basic funding for the seminar, would yield even more dividends than they had hoped when agreeing to our initial proposal.

There is an even wider background to this book. Over the past five years an emerging network of researchers and practitioners interested in the topic of communication has become loosely affiliated with the Dundee area. A number of academic publications have emerged from the work of network members, most prominently a special issue of the journal *Infant and Child Development*, entitled 'Imitation and socio-emotional processes: Implications for communicative development and interventions' (Zeedyk and Heimann 2006), but this is the first opportunity we have had to direct our collaborative efforts toward a non-academic audience. It is an occasion that delights us, given that one of the aims of the network is to utilise research knowledge in developing innovative practice. We are grateful to Jessica Kingsley Publishers, who immediately saw the potential of this volume, despite the risks presented by its unusually broad content, which meant it had no easily identifiable market.

It is important to call attention to the broader scientific context within which our network's efforts are situated. At the moment huge interest exists in communicative processes and their adaptions. In addition to the domains already touched upon, scientists are investigating whether primates create what could be called 'culture' (e.g. Tomasello 2001; Whiten in press), how marketing messages can be made even more persuasive through the incorporation of non-verbal cues (e.g. Bailenson and Yee 2005; Van Baaren *et al.* 2004), and the emotional (as opposed to cognitive) processes that underlie voters' political decisions (e.g. Schreiber 2005). Within this intellectual flurry, one of the features of social interaction that has received particular attention is imitation. Three decades ago, developmental psychologists discovered (what many parents before them must also have discovered) that newborn infants, only minutes old, were able to imitate the facial expressions of adults, including sticking out tongues or forming an 'O' shape with their mouths (Maratos 1973; Meltzoff and Moore 1977). This seemed to be an innate, biological capacity that infants possessed for connecting to other people, although controversy has continued to rumble since the 1970s about the precise functions, structures and definitions of imitation (e.g. Anisfield 1996; Heimann 2001; Kugiumutzakis 1999; Meltzoff 2002; Nadel *et al.* 1999; Nagy 2006; Zeedyk 2006). Can infants that young 'really' imitate other people? If they can be said to be 'connected' psychologically to other people, does that connection exist at the emotional, perceptual, or mental level? Could such an innate predisposition have evolutionary roots, perhaps helping parents to bond emotionally with infants and thereby ensuring they would continue to give infants care and attention?

The debate surrounding imitation has recently intensified once again, upon the discovery by an Italian team of neuroscientists of what have been dubbed 'mirror neurons' (Rizzolatti *et al.* 1995). These are neurons (i.e. cells in the brain) that seem to fire *both* when an individual performs an action and also when he or she observes that action being performed by someone else. They were discovered in the brains of primates – apparently accidentally, when the electronic recording devices implanted in the monkey's brain responded unexpectedly to the movements of one of the team members who was eating an ice cream cone. Mirror neurons have since been inferred as existing in the brains of humans. Such an overlapping function for cells, or perhaps cellular networks, implies that the connection between self and other may be so fundamental to human (and primate) functioning that it is neurally encoded. That is, interpersonal connections do not have to be learned through experience; our brains come equipped, from birth, with the ability to recognise them (Thompson 2001). The behaviours that have now been tentatively attributed to mirror neurons include yawning, the empathic identification with another person's emotions, the spontaneous copying so often observed in young children's play, the developmental imperative to acquire language, and even the experience of phantom limbs (e.g. Arbib 2005; Gallese 2006; Nadel *et al.* 2004; Ramachandran 2006; Ramachandran and Oberman 2006; Schurmann *et al.* 2005). Whether or not such proposals are eventually validated, the discovery of mirror neurons has reenergised the debate about imitation and has opened up revolutionary new spaces for the way that scientists think about human social, communicative and emotional capacities.

Evidence from the clinical and intervention literatures has much to offer this debate about the role of imitation in human functioning, even though cross-references between the basic and applied fields appear less frequently than one might expect. Empirical studies have shown that autistic children whose behaviours are imitated show unexpectedly high levels of interest in their partners (e.g. Escalona *et al.* 2002; Heimann, Laberg and Nordoen 2006; Nadel *et al.* 2000). The relationship between postnatally depressed mothers and their infants improves rapidly when mothers match their movements to those of their infants (Horowitz *et al.* 2001). Aggressive behaviour in adults with learning disabilities decreases substantially, and remains at lower levels, when staff respond to them using corresponding actions (Nind and Kellett 2002). Such findings demonstrate the need for scientists to think even more carefully about the inherent mutuality of human behaviour. Fortunately, such creative thinking is flourishing. For example, Jaak Panksepp has been for some time investigating emotions in animals as a means of better understanding human emotions (Panksepp 1998).

Ramachandran has recently speculated that many of the behaviours commonly associated with autism result from an 'autonomic storm' occluding the mirror neuron system, rather than from a fundamental disinterest in other people (Ramachandran and Oberman 2006). Alan Schore is one of many theorists now arguing that the ability of adults to read emotions in other people is grounded in the empathy that they received from others as a baby (Schore 2001; see also Sroufe *et al.* 2005; WAVE Trust 2005). These are fascinating and important avenues of investigation, for they aid not only in developing interventions to promote communicative abilities where they have become impaired in some way, but they ultimately help us to better understand the nature of our own humanity. That awareness lies at the core of the work being done by all the authors in this volume. They are each intrigued by the interconnectedness, the mutuality, that seems to be an essential component of our psychological and biological compositions as humans. A further aim for many of them is to understand how, by simply intensifying that mutuality – call the process what you will: imitation, reciprocal responsiveness, matching, speaking the other's language, attunement, affirmation – it becomes possible to transform both one's sense of connection to another human being and, simultaneously, one's sense of self.

Seeking to institute some order onto what risks becoming an amorphous agenda, the book is structured in three sections. The first section provides insights into the origins of communication. In Chapter 2 Colwyn Trevarthen begins this exploration by describing the communicative capacities that babies bring with them into the world. During his long career as a developmental psychologist Trevarthen helped to generate a cosmic shift in science's understanding of babies, for his data were among the first to show how very sensitive babies are to the behaviours of other people. His chapter traces the history of that discovery process, recalling the contributions made by a host of psychologists, brain scientists, anthropologists and others. What becomes clear is how momentous the change has been in our knowledge about the infant mind, and thus about the origins of human consciousness. We now know, for example, how important play and fun and joking are for the growth of the social brain. And we know that babies possess an innate sense of timing and rhythm, from which the human love of music derives. And we know, as Trevarthen so animatedly argues, just how misplaced traditional theories of human learning have been to assume that newborns possess only basic 'biological' abilities, maturing by merely processing information about the environment around them. It turns out that babies bring with them, from birth, the intuitive impulses with which they will make and sustain relationships, and through which the stimuli in their environment have any chance at all of coming to hold meaning for them. It is precisely these same intuitive impulses that interventions should be seeking to nurture in individuals with communicative impairments.

Raymond MacDonald develops these themes in Chapter 3, focusing on the ways in which adults retain such features within their communicative abilities. He focuses in particular on the musicality that is inherent within all adults – an awareness that arises both from his experimental research programme as a psychologist and also from his experience as a professional musician. The key point of his chapter is that music can be a particularly powerful means of connecting with other people's emotions and intentions, often outstripping the capacity of spoken language in this regard. The research programme he describes has sought to demonstrate that enhancing individuals' awareness of their musical identities supports their ability to engage with others. Thus he is essentially drawing attention to the multiple channels of communication that are often overlooked but nonetheless available to all of us, disabled and non-disabled alike.

The second section of the book examines five different ways in which communicative abilities can be impaired. In Chapter 4 Michelle O'Neill and colleagues focus on autism, a condition that alters the ways in which individuals engage socially, and one which has seen a worrying rise in prevalence over the past two decades. O'Neill reviews the literature showing that imitative responsiveness can be effective in promoting engagement, and then she describes work she has been doing, as a researcher, to teach parents to use imitative responsive techniques with their children who have autism. Her findings show that when these parents slow down and let their children take the lead in activities, using behaviours that correspond closely to the child's movements and interests, children become much more solicitous and inviting of their parents' attention. This is a major behavioural shift for these children, who are usually described as avoiding social contact. The attention to parents in O'Neill's work is particularly valuable, for consideration of family members remains oddly neglected within large sections of the autism intervention literature.

In Chapter 5, Paul Hart focuses on the domain of deafblindness. Without the ability to see and hear the world around you, it is almost impossible to learn language, right? Wrong! What Hart seeks to show, as a member of a growing movement of rather radical practitioners working in this area, is that deafblind people can develop language – it is just that theirs is based in the main sensory system available to them: touch. More specifically, speaking a tactile language becomes possible for deafblind people when, and only when, they have available to them partners who are willing to spend time exploring their 'spatial landscapes'. For with deafblind people, as with all other people, it is the mutual sharing of a landscape with other people that gives birth to representational linguistic skills. That cannot be done – there is no reason for it to be done – independently of social engagement. Hart explores the implications of this insight, both practically and theoretically. His descriptions of the interventions being developed in this field make clear that it is certainly possible (if as yet unusual) for deafblind people to tell stories about their past, plan outings for their future, and ultimately to move beyond the 'here and now' within which current practice tends to confine them. As Hart would put it, it is indeed nice to be able to ask someone for a cup of tea, but how much more invigorating to be able to recount to them, while drinking it, the story of how yesterday's teacup ended up smashed on the floor! It is such simple, but profound, theoretical insights that work in the deafblind field offers to the wider literature on communication. The work compels us to think anew about just what constitutes a 'language', how an infant manages so effortlessly to acquire one, and how the human species ever developed this astonishing capacity in the first place.

In Chapter 6 Cliff Davies and his colleagues consider a third means by which communicative processes can go awry: through severe neglect in early childhood. His research team has been working with institutionalised children in Romania, who develop autistic-like symptoms as a result of the comprehensive neglect they have experienced in state care. This team has been exploring the potential of imitative responsiveness to promote the children's interest in other people. They report here for the first time on the success of their efforts, with their outcomes suggesting that even brief training in the technique (i.e. of less than one hour) is sufficient to alter the behaviour of staff, which promptly results in an increase in the children's social engagement. Such outcomes offer positive strategies to the many regions of Eastern Europe (as well as the rest of the world) that are in the midst of trying to de-institutionalise care for abandoned and disabled children.

Pete Coia and Angela Jardine Handley turn to the domain of learning disabilities in Chapter 7. As members of the disability services within the National Health Service they have considerable experience of delivering training in communicative interventions. The point they make in their chapter is that the field should think less about 'delivery of interventions' and more about the 'forming of relationships'. All of us, whether we are labelled 'impaired' or not, frequently face challenges in ascertaining the meaning of a partner's actions. Coia and Jardine Handley have developed novel suggestions for how one could go about getting to know a new partner (or to know an old one even better!) when that process is proving challenging. Essentially, they have designed a set of 'tools' that can be called upon when an exchange feels confusing or tedious or even threatening. The refreshing message residing in their toolbox is that the process of 'getting to know you' does not have to be intuitive and spontaneous. It is perfectly acceptable to need to reach for deliberate strategies to survive the sticky stages of relationship building. Viewed from this perspective, engaging with another person becomes more about commitment than about skill.

Finally in this section, in Chapter 8, Maggie Ellis and Arlene Astell report on the exploratory work that they have been doing in the area of dementia. They have been adapting imitative interventions in order to reach elderly patients whose dementia is so far advanced that they no longer have any linguistic abilities. Such patients often suffer neglect in care homes because their social skills have become so weakened that it is easy for staff to overlook the subtle cues that they are able to display. Such disregard, even if unintentional, hastens the mental and emotional decline of these individuals. The work that Astell and Ellis are carrying out is groundbreaking. Empirically, their results demonstrate that, even at the most severe end of dementia, patients still retain the urge to communicate with others; clinically, it confirms that simple interventions can be put in place to enable staff and loved ones to nurture those abilities that do remain. This offers a more hopeful image of dementia than is commonly available, and it also provides intriguing insights into just how fundamental the capacity for communication is within human beings.

Having surveyed a range of ways in which communication can become impaired, the final section of the book focuses in more detail on interventions that can be helpful in promoting social engagement. Three different interventions are discussed: Video Interaction Guidance, Sensory Integration and Intensive Interaction. Although they have individual titles, these interventions should not be considered in any sense mutually exclusive. They could easily be used in conjunction with one another, as part of a comprehensive intervention package, largely because they operate on a shared set of principles: that to value the 'client' one must value his or her behaviour. The starting point for each of these authors is that, in order for communicative exchanges to blossom, practitioners must accept their partner's existing behaviour, seeking to understand the meaning that the behaviour holds for them. What intentions, interests, feelings does it convey? What does it provide them: comfort, reassurance, control, relief? When practitioners start from such a position of acceptance and affirmation, then unprompted, complex and often joyful exchanges quickly follow. Acts that once held isolated meaning for clients becomes shared acts for the dyad. Each of the interventions to be discussed has achieved striking outcomes by encouraging practitioners to start from the perspective of the 'other'. This approach contrasts with that of traditional behavioural approaches, which tend to be very structured, starting from a point of predetermined behavioural goals and communicative strategies that are intended for the purpose of instruction. The contributors to this volume would argue that communicative outcomes are more effective when they are mutually negotiated, requiring a style of interpersonal interaction that is necessarily spontaneous, unstructured and depends on a respect of 'intuition'. In short, people with even the most severe forms of communicative impairment remain adept at and eager for free-flowing conversation; they just need the rest of us, their partners, to be willing to listen more carefully.

In Chapter 9 Hilary Kennedy and Heather Sked discuss the intervention of Video Interaction Guidance, which was initially developed in the Netherlands in the 1980s, and has since been used widely throughout the UK. The aim of Video Interaction Guidance is to facilitate engagement between two (or more) people, focusing on the positive, intersubjective elements that already exist within an interaction. It insists on a collaborative, empowering relationship between coach and client, with the focus always kept on future potential, rather than current failings. Amongst other contexts, it has been used to support interactions between parents and infants, teachers and pupils, health professionals and patients and, as described in detail in this chapter, special needs auxiliary workers and autistic children. As educational psychologists, Kennedy and Sked are well aware of the difficulty of dislodging hierarchy from the classroom, but their central point is that when one begins from a position of collaboration, then new motivational vistas open up for both partners. The traditionally powerful partner finds his or her drive, confidence and compassion renewed; the traditionally subordinate partner displays more initiative, interest and ability than may ever have been predicted for him or her. These values fit with the paradigm shift that seems to be under way within the educational and parenting literatures, which are increasingly emphasising the importance of creative relationships for achieving whatever curriculum outcomes are desired. The hope of Kennedy and Sked is that Video Interaction Guidance is recognised as one practical means of pioneering such relationships.

Jane Horwood in Chapter 10 then describes her experiences, as an occupational therapist, of using the intervention of Sensory Integration. This approach developed, like so many of the other interventions discussed in this book, during the 1970s and 1980s, and has subsequently garnered attention in various regions throughout the world and from various professional sectors (e.g. paediatrics, learning disabilities, mental health). The main aim of Sensory Integration is to draw attention to the multiple ways in which sensory experience underwrites and frames all human activity. For example, Horwood describes the way in which children may go into 'sensory meltdown' as staff unwittingly try to coax them out of the corner in which they feel safe and prevent them from engaging in the rocking that is calming their vestibular system. Thinking about behaviour from a 'sensory point of view' transforms the way one interprets another's actions. Resistance can now be seen as fear, disinterest as confusion, aggression as self-protection. Staff begin to feel less confused and frustrated; it is easier for them to find a compassionate and creative means of helping those they work with to achieve the tasks facing them – whether that is getting a spoon of food into their mouth, coming back inside after playtime or focusing on academic assignments. One of the jewels of Horwood's account is that she makes vividly clear how all of us are affected by sensory stimulation. Some of us can't stand the itchy tag at the back of a new shirt, others of us wouldn't go near a theme park ride, and then there are those of us who can't possibly relax until the dinner dishes are washed up and tidied away. The many tips that Horwood offers for supporting sensory integration become, therefore, more than practical suggestions for working with communicatively impaired individuals. They become a means through which all of us can boost our own self-awareness and our empathy for others.

Finally, in Chapter 11, Phoebe Caldwell discusses the intervention of Intensive Interaction, which has been widely used throughout the UK in working with people with learning disabilities or autism, especially where their condition is accompanied by distressed behaviour. While several other chapters in the book also deal with Intensive Interaction, Caldwell's chapter offers the most comprehensive explanation as to why matching a partner's movements and rhythms should serve as such a powerful means of fostering engagement. As one of the leading Intensive Interaction practitioners in the country, she is well placed to offer this theoretical account. The case study she presents of a child with severe autism illustrates how rapidly this approach is able to reach withdrawn individuals, and how moving that union is for both partners. Such an outcome, unpredicted by contemporary theories of autism, encourages a rethink about the way in which autism is currently explained and treated. Caldwell would go as far as arguing that, rather than being unmindful of social cues, autistic individuals are hypersensitive to them. This represents a major conceptual shift from contemporary mainstream views of autism. This is an example of 'applied work' at its best: achieving practical outcomes for clients' lives, while opening up new sites for theoretical deliberation.

Our hope in creating this volume was to give some sense of the insights that stand to be gained from examining human communication interdisciplinarily. Challenges that once seemed intractable when viewed from within a familiar domain can dissolve when viewed from a wider perspective. Science is revealing, with increasingly sophisticated technology, the deep-seated mutuality of human experience. It seems that, even at the neural level, as the brain engages with the body, human beings are psychologically connected to one another. This collection of papers makes clear that not only do practitioners and family members stand to benefit from these insights, via new intervention techniques, but that their observations can also play a key role in determining the theoretical questions that need next to be asked. It bodes well that the experience of these authors is that, however severe the communicative impairment, it is always possible to find some way of making contact.

References

Anisfield, M. (1996) 'Only tongue protrusion modelling is matched by neonates.' *Developmental Review 16*, 149–161.

Arbib, M.A. (2005) 'From monkey-like action recognition to human language: An evolutionary framework for neurolinguistics.' *Behavioural and Brain Sciences 28*, 105–124.

Bailenson, J.N. and Yee, N. (2005) 'Digital chameleons: Automatic assimilation of nonverbal gestures in immersive virtual environments.' *Psychological Science 16*, 814–819.

Escalona, A., Field, T., Nadel, J. and Lundy, B. (2002) 'Brief report: Imitation effects on children with autism.' *Journal of Autism and Developmental Disorders 32*, 141–144.

Gallese, V. (2006) 'Mirror neurons and intentional attunement: Commentary of Olds.' *Journal of the American Psychoanalytic Association 54*, 47–57.

Heimann, M. (2001) 'Neonatal Imitation – A Fuzzy Phenomenon?' In F. Lacerda, C. von Hofsten and M. Heimann (eds) *Emerging Cognitive Abilities in Early Infancy*. London: Lawrence Erlbaum Associates.

Heimann, M., Laberg, K.E. and Nordoen, B. (2006) 'Imitative interaction increases social interest and elicited imitation in non-verbal children with autism.' *Infant and Child Development 15*, 297–309.

Horowitz, J.A., Bell, M., Trybulski, J., Munro, B.H. *et al.* (2001) 'Promoting responsiveness between mothers with depressive symptoms and their infants.' *Journal of Nursing Scholarship 33*, 323–329.

Kugiumutzakis, G. (1999) 'Genesis and Development of Early Infant Mimesis to Facial and Vocal Models.' In J. Nadel and G. Butterworth (eds) *Imitation in Infancy*. Cambridge: Cambridge University Press.

Maratos, O. (1973) 'The origin and development of imitation in the first six months of life.' PhD thesis, University of Geneva.

Meltzoff, A.N. (2002) 'Elements of a Developmental Theory of Imitation.' In A.N. Meltzoff and W. Prinz (eds) *The Imitative Mind: Development, Evolution, and Brain Bases*. Cambridge: Cambridge University Press.

Meltzoff, A.N. and Moore, M.K. (1977) 'Imitation of facial and manual gestures by newborn infants.' *Science 198*, 75–78.

Nadel, J., Croue, S., Mattlinger, M.J., Canet, P. *et al.* (2000) 'Do children with autism have expectancies about the social behaviour of unfamiliar people?' *Autism 4*, 133–145.

Nadel, J., Guerini, C., Peze, A. and Rivet, C. (1999) 'The Evolving Nature of Imitation as a Transitory Means of Communication.' In J. Nadel and G. Butterworth (eds) *Imitation in Infancy*. Cambridge: Cambridge University Press.

Nadel, J., Revel, A. Andry, P. and Gaussier, P. (2004) 'Toward communication: First imitation in infants, low-functioning children with autism and robots.' *Interaction Studies 5*, 45–74.

Nagy, E. (2006) 'From imitation to conversation: The first dialogues with human neonates.' *Infant and Child Development 15*, 223–232.

National Literacy Trust (2007) 'Talk to your baby campaign.' Accessed on 1/11/07 at www.literarytrust.org.uk.

Nind, M. and Kellett, M. (2002) 'Responding to individuals with severe learning difficulties and stereotyped behaviour: Challenges for an inclusive era.' *European Journal of Special Needs Education 3*, 265–282.

Panksepp, J. (1998) *Affective Neuroscience: The Foundations of Human and Animal Emotions.* Oxford: Oxford University Press.

Parsons, S. and Mitchell, P. (2002) 'The potential of virtual reality in social skills training for people with autistic spectrum disorders.' *Journal of Intellectual Disability Research 4*, 6, 430–443.

Rage Against the Darkness (2004) Television film by J. Kastner. Accessed on 1/11/07 at www.jskastner.com/.

Ramachandran, V.S. (2006) 'The Uniqueness of the Human Brain.' Film. http://video.google.com/videoplay?docid=-4684607596399338611; www.almaden.ibm.com.

Ramachandran, V.S. and Oberman, L.M. (2006) 'Broken mirrors: A theory of autism.' *Scientific American 295* (November), 39–45.

Rizzolatti, G., Camarda, R., Gallese, V. and Fogassi, L. (1995) 'Premotor cortex and the recognition of motor actions.' *Cognitive Brain Research 3*, 131–141.

Schore, A.N. (2001) 'Effects of a secure attachment relationship on right-brain development, affect regulation, and infant mental health.' *Infant Mental Health Journal 22*, 7–66.

Schreiber, D. (2005) 'Monkey see, monkey do: Mirror neurons, functional brain imaging, and looking at political faces.' Paper presented at the Annual Meeting of the American Political Science Association, Washington DC. Accessed on 1/11/07 at www.all-academic.com/meta/p40055_index.html.

Schurmann, M., Hesse, M.D., Stephan, K.E., Saarela, M. *et al.* (2005) 'Yearning to yawn: the neural basis of contagious yawning.' *Neuroimage 24*, 1260–1264.

Sroufe, L.A., Egeland, B., Carlson, E.A. and Collins, W.A. (2005) 'Placing Early Attachment Experiences in Developmental Context: The Minnesota Longitudinal Study.' In K.E. Grossmann, K. Grossman and E. Waters (eds) *Attachment from Infancy to Adulthood.* New York: Guildford Press.

Thompson, E. (2001) 'Empathy and consciousness.' *Journal of Consciousness Studies 8*, 5–7, 1–32.

Tomasello, M. (2001) 'Cultural transmission: A view from chimpanzees and human infants.' *Journal of Cross-Cultural Psychology 31*, 135–156.

Van Baaren, R.B. (2005) 'The parrot effect: How to increase tip size.' *Cornell Hotel and Restaurant Administration Quarterly 46*, 79–84.

Van Baaren, R.B., Holland, R.W., Kawakami, K. and van Knippenberg, A. (2004) 'Mimicry and prosocial behaviour.' *Psychological Science 15*, 71–74.

WAVE Trust (2005) *The WAVE Report 2005: Violence and What To Do About It.* London: Wave Trust. Accessed on 1/11/07 at www.wavetrust.org.

Whiten, A. (in press) 'The Identification of Culture in Chimpanzees and Other Animals: From Natural History to Diffusion Experiments.' In K.N. Laland and B.G. Galef (eds) *The Question of Animal Culture.* Cambridge, MA: Harvard University Press.

Zeedyk, M.S. (2006) 'From intersubjectivity to subjectivity: The transformative roles of emotional intimacy and imitation.' *Infant and Child Development 15,* 321–344.

Zeedyk, M.S. and Heimann, M. (eds) (2006) 'Imitation and socio-emotional processes: Implications for communicative development and interventions.' *Infant and Child Development 15* (special issue), 219–344.

PART I

Origins of Communication

CHAPTER 2

INTUITION FOR HUMAN COMMUNICATION

Colwyn Trevarthen

Human beings are born to be sociable. All infants enter the world already able to communicate, to share experience. A wealth of studies conducted over the past four decades have revealed just how sophisticated babies' social capacities are. This realisation has implications across a wide range of domains: for interpreting the brain and physiological development, for understanding the influence of early parenting styles and the cultural mismatch that accompanies immigration, and for perceiving and assisting 'developmental disorders' such as autism or the effects of neglect or abuse. I will bring together some of these themes by describing how very sensitive human beings of all ages are to the 'musicality' of one another's movements, how this sensitivity is active even from moments after birth, and how the project of infant development unfolds within sympathetic companionship. These abilities for 'communicative musicality' have a clear message for people seeking to communicate with individuals of any age who have communicative impairments.

I offer these observations as a biologist and brain scientist who, for the past 40 years, has chosen to look closely at how infants communicate and learn. I have learned how to use recordings of natural communications between babies and toddlers and their parents to get evidence about the motives in brains that drive consciousness and the development of relationships, communication and knowledge. I will summarise what I think are the main findings of this large body of work, because I believe this can assist psychologists and health care professionals who, like the many authors in this volume, want to help people with communicative impairments to have richer, happier lives supported by companions who understand them.

Why we learn, and what we all know in order to do it

In our industrious technical culture, life seems to depend entirely on skills and knowledge learned. Teaching in school is necessary for success in life, and the skills and knowledge children have to learn are spelled out and tested. Being able to speak well, and then to read, write and calculate are regarded as 'basic', and now a young person is expected to become fluent in the endlessly multiplying and varied forms of 'information' carried by e-media. A toddler's doll is now likely to 'be', and move and talk, on a cell phone. The human mind seems to be thought of as a great sponge that absorbs facts that make it clever at doing and making things, or a great notebook with many blank sheets on which life experiences are to be written. Our governments are concerned that every child should be instructed in the proper ways to communicate and work in complex social communities, institutions and businesses. Any person who does not easily acquire the right skills or techniques is classed as handicapped, with 'special needs'. What people cannot do is carefully diagnosed, and they are given special training to make up for their inability to learn as others can.

And yet we are not just receivers of knowledge. All human beings, even the most handicapped, can respond sensitively and with their own initiative to expressions of other persons, provided these persons are sympathetic. We all could move in subtle ways and communicate with an affectionate mother immediately after birth. Something is wrong with the view of human intelligence as that which is learned, and the view of human personality as a set of limitations on possible learning. Innate, intuitive powers of the mind, in a brain that moves the thousands of muscles in the body with such sensitive awareness of what will happen, are not properly understood by a psychology that accepts a model of consciousness, intelligence and personality that focuses only on the cognitive processing of information.

There are changes happening in the way scientists are thinking about the mind, and these depend on two kinds of discovery that seem to grant the inside of human nature more importance. A richer, more 'common sense' philosophy of mind is gaining ground. In the past 40 years there have been very surprising findings from careful observation of what children are born able to do, and how they develop understanding with companions before they can talk. Then, more recently, research on activity in the brains of animals and people has proved that the source of consciousness is in what is generated to make sense of experience – the intentions and expected risks and benefits of what the environment will offer. Most importantly, the intentions to move the body have immediate communicative power. Animal brains reflect or resonate to the emotionally expressive forms and intended directions of looking, listening, smelling, tasting and touching that show what individuals want to do, what they expect will happen, and how they feel about it. Brains, by means of bodies, communicate purposes, interests, concerns and feelings by an intuitive unlearned process, one that links individuals within intimate relationships and that regulates a social community. All learning depends on these unlearned motives. That is how human culture works, too.

The new intentional and affective psychology gives a different and much richer appreciation of the newborn baby's mind and how developments in infancy motivate the learning of others' meanings. It also explains how engaging sensitively with even the most intellectually or physically handicapped persons, be they damaged by faults in development, injured by accidents of life or illness, or just very old, can release real communication and bring pleasure from companionship. Every live human person has some of this intuitive capacity to share intentions and feelings, and to make friends.

Discovering motives, principles and emotions of communication before language

Important evidence for the science of human communication came in the late 1960s from infancy research. The time was ripe for several of us to reject the view prevailing at the time that infants are mindless organisms driven by stimuli, and adapted merely for eliciting care for their vital bodily needs. Close observation of engagements between infants and their mothers found proof that there is an intuitive sharing of complex, dynamic states of mind, made evident and interesting by special expressive movement of the body. These earliest communications were very human.

An anthropologist and linguist, Mary Catherine Bateson (1979), studied a film of a nine-week-old baby 'chatting' with the mother, and she called what she observed 'protoconversation', which she concluded was the foundation, not only for language, but for 'ritual healing practices that use rhythm, intonation and repetition to promote social engagement, and a sense of being part of the community in someone who is ill or mentally distressed. Child psychiatrist Daniel Stern (1971) analysed a recording of a mother playing with three-month-old twins and he saw musical, dancing forms of joking and teasing with a mutually regulated rhythm. This led him to greatly extend ideas of psychoanalysis about how human engagements and self-awareness are formed, and to lead the way in formulating a theory of the 'interpersonal world' of infancy. Stern collaborated with experts on adult dialogue dynamics, and this team showed that dialogues of mothers and infants had the same regularities, in timing and turn taking, as those of adults, thus showing how skilled mother and infant each are.

In the Harvard Center for Cognitive Studies, set up for infancy research by Jerome Bruner, a group of us set out to make film recordings of mothers and babies (Brazelton, Koslowski and Main 1974; Bruner 1968; Richards 1973; Trevarthen 1974). This team included Berry Brazelton, a paediatrician, Martin Richards, an animal ethologist who had been studying maternal care in hamsters, and myself. We made the recordings in a set-up where we could observe in detail what the mother and baby each did and could study the to-and-fro of expressions as the two played. We saw the same conversational games that Bateson had identified, and noted they were well established by six weeks, and we followed transformations in the babies' interests in people and things after three months as well as the effects on the mother's playfulness, her use of expressive movements and language, and the sharing of interest in objects that drew the babies' curiosity and attempts at possession. I was convinced that a careful study of age-related developments before language was needed, and that the infants' intuitive skills were regulating the changes, with the mother's sympathetic support. Both were clever at this primary communication, and both could guide its development to more elaborate cooperative forms.

After 1971 at Edinburgh University, this project, to trace developments week by week through the first year, was put into effect and we charted systematic changes in infants' motives that led through ritual games with communicative expressions and objects to cooperation in shared tasks, a clear prerequisite for learning the meanings of words to describe intended actions and their goals. A very important study of the emotions that regulate early dialogues with infants was set up by Lynne Murray (Murray and Trevarthen 1985). She showed that if the mother failed to show well-timed sympathetic emotional reactions to her infant's expressions of interest in her and pleasure in sharing, this would

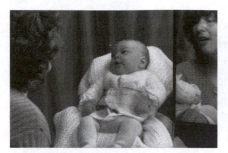

Figure 2.1: Laura, six weeks old, in the Infant Communication Lab., Edinburgh in 1979. She looks intently and coos to her mother, who listens and is ready to imitate in reply.

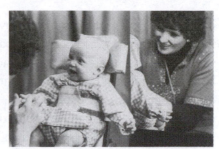

Figure 2.2: Leanne, at five months, watches her mother eagerly as she recites, 'Round and round the garden, like a teddy bear.' Leanne knows the verse and vocalises in tune with her mother on the final rhyming vowel '…and a tickly under THERE.'

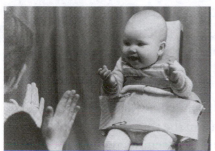

Figure 2.3: Emma, six months old, is very happy learning 'Clappa, clappa, handies' with her mother, in the Lab.

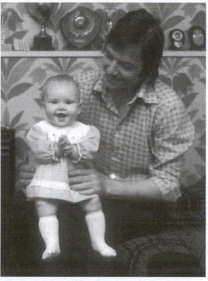

Figure 2.4: At home Emma is proud to show the photographer how she can clap, when her mother asks her to 'Clap handies!'

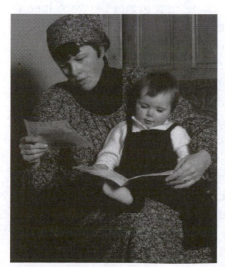

Figure 2.5: Basilie, one year old, reads her book at home, while her mother reads a telephone bill.

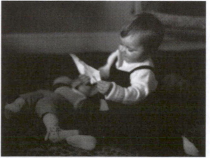

Figure 2.6: Then she happily reads her mother's mail, with a 'busy' manner, making 'important' talking sounds.

immediately cause the infant to show behaviours of withdrawal and distress. The infant was seeking a particular quality of commitment to sharing actions and experiences, and this sharing was powerfully regulated by what Stern later named 'relational emotions', not just named 'categorical emotions' of happiness, sadness, anger, etc. Lynne later applied what she had learned to the study of the effects of a mother's postnatal depression on the infant's state of mind and cognitive development (Murray 1992), a field in which she is now a leading authority.

A decade before the discoveries made in the 1960s John Bowlby (1958) had called for a transformation of hospital care for infants and their mothers on the basis of his observations of the devastating effects that deprivation of maternal care could have in the first year of a baby's life. His formulation of Attachment Theory has become the foundation for most clinical appraisal and treatment of affective and learning disorders following from poor support through infancy. Research by Mary Ainsworth (Ainsworth and Bell 1970) showed that the immediate effects of insensitive mothering (in its various forms) could be recorded and measured, and these measures were related to outcomes in the development of children. At the same time it was clear from the studies of play that infants have needs for more than just sensitive protection and care. Important developments in care for infants who had seriously troubled beginnings were developed by clinicians, and these included realisations of the importance of play and its creativity.

Careful observations of intuitive 'chats' and games between infants and adults have proved that infants see and hear what is motivating our looks, facial expressions, vocalisations and hand gestures, and that they want to engage. A baby can imitate our body signs from immediately after birth, and this imitation is not automatic or a mechanical reproduction of a movement, but rather a bid for an exchange, an invitation or a comment. Right from the start it is coloured by emotions of interest and pleasure, or by puzzlement and disappointment if the response is not as intuitively predicted. The Greek psychologist Giannis Kugiumutzakis has insisted for many years that imitation is not just a form of learning, but an emotion-charged act of communication (Kugiumutzakis 1998).

As the baby becomes stronger and more alert to the many events around, so communication becomes more lively or playful. The baby starts to enjoy what Vasu Reddy (1991, 2003, 2005) calls 'joking, teasing and mucking about'. Guessing what the other will do in teasing is fun, as long as attention is paid to the feelings of the other and the game does not become 'mean'. Animals enjoy play fighting or rough and tumble play, and the scientist of emotional systems in the brain, Jaak Panksepp, who discovered that playing rats 'laugh', thinks that enjoying play with companions is the way the social brain grows (Panksepp 2005, 2007). All good communication has a touch of playfulness. Fun does the brain good.

But play with human infants develops a special creativity and message power. Infants are attracted to extended engagement with human voice and gestures, while sympathetic to many emotions – resonating to the impulses and qualities of movement; imitating; seeking an active part in protoconversations or playful duets of agency. When the expressive forms are examined in detail, infant and partner are found to be sharing a subtle 'musicality' of communication.

Rhythm and sympathy: The essential 'communicative musicality' of human motives and the 'time of life'

Experiments by Sandra Trehub (1990) and colleagues testing infants' listening found surprising evidence that they have a delicate sensitivity for musical features of a mother's voice or, indeed, for the kinds of sounds made by instruments, detecting pulse, rhythms, pitch, harmony and melodies. Obviously these listening skills are adapted from early infancy for communication of feelings and interests, especially with the mother. Mechthild and Hanuš Papoušek (1981) compared the musical features of the vocalisations of their daughters to the sounds of parents' speech to infants, and they concluded that their correspondence indicated that musical talk to infants paves the way for learning the parents' language. Ellen Dissanayake (2000) finds this intimate communication to be the source of art, most obviously musical, poetic or dramatic art, making special stories of human interest. Very soon the early baby songs and action games, which have similar expressive temporal and melodic features across languages, containing comparable rhythms, phrases and verses or stanzas, become the habits or conventions of what Maya Gratier (2003) calls a mini-culture. For each pair of mother and child, these improvised creations of meaning become treasured memories of a special relationship. Babies over four months old learn songs and games quickly, and may move in rhythm to sounds of music, sometimes trying to sing.

Perhaps the most stimulating part of our new thinking about the infant mind as 'musical' is the abundant evidence that humans have an innate sense of time for moving in expressive ways, and for sharing it. Infants, even as they are still growing their bodies and learning to use them well, sense an inner 'time in the mind' well from the start. They get in rhythm with other persons, creating what Dan Stern (1999) named 'narratives of feelings'. This has stimulated a new science of 'communicative musicality'. The 'meaning' of music has been made clear by this innate sense of shared rhythm, expressive gesture, and phrasing, and this discovery changes the way we think about the learning of language and other skills of culture. As the Danish Jazz player and music psychologist Ole Kühl put it, 'What we share in music is not just sound, but also, and perhaps more importantly, time. We share structured time, when we share music. When we hear music, we entrain to a pulse, while we synchronise ourselves cognitively to a temporal pattern of expectations and predictions, set up through musical form and gestures' (Kühl 2007, p.25).

People of all ages and all levels of education express their inner time for moving in everything they do: in breath; in the beating of the heart; walking in different tempi from deeply thoughtful or sorrowful *largo*, to casual strolling *andante*, lively *allegro* or hurrying *presto*; in grasping and manipulating things and in gesturing thoughts and feeling; in speaking; and in singing or playing a musical instrument. It not only sets up trains of pulses with different energy – it frames phrases, and gives narrative form to longer communications, building from *introduction* through *development* to a *climax* of meaning in excitement, then falling back to rest in a *resolution*. This inner time and its mini dramas is immediately communicated when brains, linked by bodies and their senses, synchronise and resonate in sympathy. Every rhythmic gesture has a quality of urgency or restraint that communicates the feeling that generated it. This interpersonal traffic of time and expression in movement is the foundation for all communication, from its beginnings and in all applications, from casual conversation to teaching and learning and in therapy. It animates shared consciousness between mother and infant in what Peter Hobson (2002) calls 'the cradle of thought'. It makes it possible for traditions of meaning to be built up and passed from generation to generation. The Norwegian musicologist Jon-Roar Bjørkvold (1992) has recorded how, from the rhythms and sounds of play, in their dancing and singing, children in Russia, the United States and Norway create their own 'musical culture', using an enormous range of musical sensibilities.

Problems from the 'cognitive revolution' and support from brain science

I believe the new awareness of human motives and their creativity, gained by observations of intuitive processes of human companionship in infancy and through childhood, must be reasserted. Current technical developments in media, recreation and teaching favour a rational science of human beings as processors of information or biomechanical systems that function like our more ingenious tools, especially those without bodies and brains that simulate calculations, or that formulate the inferences and the rules of informative language in text.

Happily the new exploratory science of the brain has produced evidence that is paradoxical for this technical 'informatics' of human initiative. There is a responsibility now to admit a psychology of sympathy or a neuroscience of 'basic trust'. For with this – the observation of how infants take an active part in participant learning of cultural rituals, techniques and arts before they speak – we may gain a better appreciation of how to support both experience and wellbeing in communication with persons of any age with impairments in their moving and perceiving. We can give proper attention to sharing their initiatives and supporting their intuitions.

Implications for communicating with persons who have impairments – for aiding their intuitive impulses

The Russian scholar of literature and educational psychologist, Lev Semenovich Vygotsky, became interested in communication to aid children with impairments in their awareness or mobility. He defined a 'zone of proximal development' as the region in which a teacher aids the aspirations of a pupil by adding to his or her efforts in helpful ways (Vygotsky 1967). Barbara Rogoff (2003) finds that in many cultures there is little or no school, and a form of apprenticeship in skills or 'intent participation learning', in which adult and child share meaningful and useful tasks, is how children become skilled and respected contributors to the culture of their community. That is, teaching occurs by supporting and extending the learner's *intuition*, not by instructing according to someone else's agenda or curriculum. The same belief in engagement with motives for learning is applied where a music therapist 'improvises' new powers of communication with a client, according to the method of Paul Nordoff

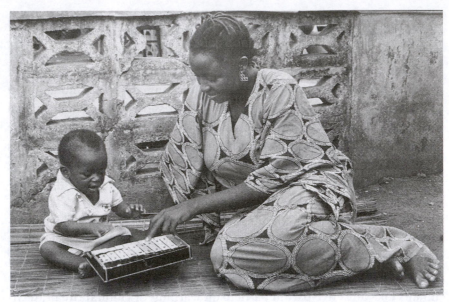

Figure 2.7: In Lagos, Nigeria, one-year-old Adegbenro gets a piano lesson from his mother, who fits with his interest.

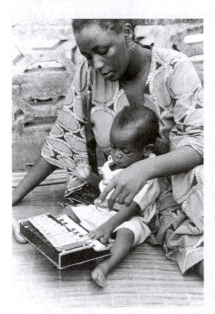

Figure 2.8: Adegbenro takes over.

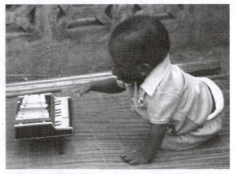

Figure 2.9: He can play and sing on his own.

(Photographs by John and Penelope Hubley, 1980.)

and Clive Robbins (2007). In these methods of education one human agent enters into collaboration with the *intentions* of another, assisting the latter to a higher level of skill, motivation or emotional regulation.

Musical sounds, especially those resembling the mother's voice, can calm distress of a newborn, giving rhythm to delicate life. It has been proved that in the last two months of gestation a foetus inside the mother's body can hear and learn the individual features of the mother's speaking or singing voice, and there is evidence that an emotional state of stress transmitted to the foetus by hormonal changes, movements or sounds of the mother's body can affect the developing brain. Our biology has adapted us for sharing both vital processes inside the body and the intentions, interests and feelings of mental life in engagement with the world.

It is of great interest to a psychobiologist such as myself that the simple form of narrative we have found in natural mother–infant protoconversations and baby songs has a period of around 20 to 40 seconds. In a very lively song, like 'Jack and Jill went up the hill' the whole little story will be finished in 15 seconds. If you recite 'Rock a bye baby, on the tree top. When the wind blows, the cradle will rock. When the bough breaks, the cradle will fall. Down will come baby, cradle and all!' in a natural way, as a lullaby, this little drama, which a five-month-old can learn, will take about 30 seconds. This time of about half a minute coincides with the interval found in studies of 'cardiac vagal tone' that record the cycles of heartbeat linked to breathing in people when they are sleeping, which in turn are coupled to bursts of nerve tissue activity that may be consolidating memories in the brain. Clearly the regulated vital states of the body are part of the process of mental integration, and they also pace the self-expression that mediates in the communication of awareness and emotions between persons of any age. When baby and mother share the stories of their mutual interest, they are coupling the movements of body and soul with this rhythm. They are sharing what Ed Tronick (2005) calls 'dyadic regulation of psychobiological states'.

For mental health or happiness a person must keep a balance between the inevitable, and often enjoyable, stress of being active and the rest that is essential for recuperation of strength. Memories and imaginary situations and events activate mechanisms stimulating activity. The stress or costs that those activities might entail must be estimated. Learned anticipations of pleasure or of painful stress are communicated between us as we share experiences, purposes and emotions. Thus, people cooperate in

sharing both effort and the pleasure of relaxing. This, as Csikszentmihalyi and Csikszentmihalyi (1988) explain, enables human beings to
find enthusiasm for great and small actions, both inventively and cooper-
atively, in the 'flow' of optimal experience. But memories or imagined
events also open the way for trauma and retention of weakness or suffer-
ing associated with particular places, events or persons. Reforming a
person's assessment of risk and rebuilding their self-confidence in psychotherapy depends on the proper management of the dynamic balance
of slow processes of autonomic and mental change in narrative time
periods, outside the immediate conscious present. The therapist has to
become a supportive part of the process that motivates rewarding experience, by seeking to be in tune with the patient's interests, wishes, enthusi-
asms and intuitions.

The discoveries about the endowments of infants for intimate emotional relationships and for learning friendships, and their emotional
needs for sympathetic companionship, were adopted after the 1970s by
clinicians. John Bowlby's observations of the distress and depression of
infants separated from their mothers, along with the Neonatal Behavioral
Assessment Scale (NBAS) developed in 1973 by Berry Brazelton and his
colleagues, transformed hospital care of newborns and infants, and
changed attitudes concerning the role of the mother at home. The NBAS
provides help to parents, health care providers and researchers to understand the newborn's 'language'. 'The Scale gives us the chance to see
what the baby's behavior will tell us,' says Dr Brazelton, Professor Emeritus, Harvard Medical School. 'It gives us a window into what it will take
to nurture the baby.' In 1980 Selma Fraiberg, a social worker, introduced
a concept of 'infant mental health' that was revolutionary for psychiatry,
as it had been assumed that infants could not have complex psychological
needs or, consequently, mental illness. Then Lynne Murray (1992),
Tiffany Field (1992) and Ed Tronick (Tronick and Field 1986; Tronick
and Weinberg 1997) presented evidence that the baby of a depressed
mother can develop a clinical depression that impairs development.
These understandings of the early stages of human sensibility and capacities for psychological communication are relevant to all ages, for the core
relational processes are innate, and they remain available to animate pur-
poseful awareness and all engagements with other persons and their
minds, actions and feelings.

The goal and function of all human communication is to discover meaning in the infinitely rich possibilities of shared intuition. All human beings, even the youngest, the oldest and the most impaired in capacities of communication, retain motives to find and share meaning.

References

Ainsworth, M.D.S. and Bell, S. (1970) 'Attachment, exploration, and separation illustrated by the behavior of one-year-olds in a strange situation.' *Child Development 41*, 49–67.

Bateson, M.C. (1979) 'The Epigenesis of Conversational Interaction: A Personal Account of Research Development.' In M. Bullowa (ed.) *Before Speech: The Beginning of Human Communication.* Cambridge: Cambridge University Press.

Bjørkvold, J.-R. (1992) *The Muse Within: Creativity and Communication, Song and Play from Childhood through Maturity.* New York: Harper Collins.

Bowlby, J. (1958) 'The nature of the child's tie to his mother.' *International Journal of Psychoanalysis 39*, 1–23.

Brazelton, T.B. (1973) *Neonatal Behavioural Assessment Scale* (Clinics in Developmental Medicine, 50. Spastics International Medical Publications). London: Heinemann Medical Books. Accessed on 2/11/07 at www.brazelton-institute.com/intro.html.

Brazelton, T.B. (1993) *Touchpoints: Your Child's Emotional and Behavioral Development.* New York: Viking.

Brazelton, T.B., Koslowski, B. and Main, M. (1974) 'The Origins of Reciprocity: The Early Mother–Infant Interaction.' In M. Lewis and L.A. Rosenblum (eds) *The Effect of the Infant on its Caregiver.* New York/London: Wiley.

Bruner, J.S. (1968) *Processes of Cognitive Growth: Infancy.* (Heinz Werner Lectures, 1968) Worcester, MA: Clark University Press with Barri Publishers.

Csikszentmihalyi, M. and Csikszentmihalyi, I.S. (eds) (1988) *Optimal Experience: Psychological Studies of Flow in Consciousness.* New York: Cambridge University Press.

Dissanayake, E. (2000) *Art and Intimacy: How the Arts Began.* University of Washington Press, Seattle and London.

Field, T.M. (1992) 'Infants of depressed mothers.' *Development and Psychopathology 4*, 49–66.

Fraiberg, S. (1980) *Clinical Studies in Infant Mental Health: The First Year of Life.* London: Tavistock.

Gratier, M. (2003) 'Expressive timing and interactional synchrony between mothers and infants: Cultural similarities, cultural differences, and the immigration experience.' *Cognitive Development 18*, 533–554.

Hobson, P. (2002) *The Cradle of Thought: Exploring the Origins of Thinking.* London: Macmillan.

Kugiumutzakis, G. (1998) 'Neonatal Imitation in the Intersubjective Companion Space.' In S. Bråten (ed.) *Intersubjective Communication and Emotion in Early Ontogeny.* Cambridge: Cambridge University Press.

Kugiumutzakis, G., Kokkinaki, T. Markodimitraki, M. and Vitalaki, E. (2005) 'Emotions in Early Mimesis.' In J. Nadel and D. Muir (eds) *Emotional Development*. Oxford: Oxford University Press.

Kühl, O. (2007) *Musical Semantics* (European Semiotics: Language, Cognition and Culture, No. 7). Bern: Peter Lang.

Murray, L. (1992) 'The impact of postnatal depression on infant development.' *Journal of Child Psychology and Psychiatry 33*, 3, 543–561.

Murray, L. and Trevarthen, C. (1985) 'Emotional Regulation of Interactions Between Two-month-olds and their Mothers.' In T.M. Field and N.A. Fox (eds) *Social Perception in Infants*. Norwood, NJ: Ablex.

Nordoff, P. and Robbins, C. (2007) *Creative Music Therapy: A Guide to Fostering Clinical Musicianship*, rev. ed. Gilsum, NH: Barcelona Publishers.

Panksepp, J. (2005) 'Beyond a joke: From animal laughter to human joy?' *Science 308*, 62–63

Panksepp, J. (2007) 'Can PLAY diminish ADHD and facilitate the construction of the social brain?' *Journal of the Canadian Academy of Child and Adolescent Psychiatry 16*, 2, 5–14.

Papoušek, M. and Papoušek, H. (1981) 'Musical Elements in the Infant's Vocalization: Their Significance for Communication, Cognition, and Creativity.' In L.P. Lipsitt and C.K. Rovee-Collier (eds) *Advances in Infancy Research, Vol. 1*. Norwood, NJ: Ablex.

Reddy, V. (1991) 'Playing with Others' Expectations: Teasing and Mucking about in the First Year.' In A. Whiten (ed.) *Natural Theories of Mind: Evolution, Development and Simulation of Everyday Mindreading*. Oxford: Blackwell.

Reddy, V. (2003) 'On being the object of attention: Implications for self–other consciousness.' *TRENDS in Cognitive Sciences 7*, 9, 397–402.

Reddy, V. (2005) 'Feeling Shy and Showing-off: Self-conscious Emotions Must Regulate Self-awareness.' In J. Nadel and D. Muir (eds) *Emotional Development*. Oxford: Oxford University Press.

Richards, M.P.M. (1973) 'The Development of Psychological Communication in the First Year of Life.' In J.S. Bruner and F.J. Connolly (eds) *The Growth of Competence*. London and New York: Academic Press.

Rogoff, B. (2003) *The Cultural Nature of Human Development*. Oxford: OUP.

Stern, D.N. (1971) 'A micro-analysis of mother-infant interaction: Behaviors regulating social contact between a mother and her three-and-a-half-month-old twins.' *Journal of American Academy of Child Psychiatry 10*, 501–517.

Stern, D.N. (1999) 'Vitality Contours: The Temporal Contour of Feelings as a Basic Unit for Constructing the Infant's Social Experience.' In P. Rochat (ed.) *Early Social Cognition: Understanding Others in the First Months of Life*. Mahwah, NJ: Erlbaum.

Trehub, S.E. (1990) 'The Perception of Musical Patterns by Human Infants: The Provision of Similar Patterns by their Parents.' In M.A. Berkley and W.C. Stebbins (eds) *Comparative Perception: Vol. 1*. Basic Mechanisms. New York: Wiley.

Trevarthen, C. (1974) 'The psychobiology of speech development.' In E.H. Lenneberg (ed) 'Language and brain: Developmental aspects.' *Neurosciences Research Program Bulletin*, 12, 570–585.

Tronick, E.Z. (2005) 'Why is Connection with Others so Critical? The Formation of Dyadic States of Consciousness: Coherence Governed Selection and the Co-creation of Meaning out of Messy Meaning Making.' In J. Nadel and D. Muir (eds) *Emotional Development*. Oxford: Oxford University Press.

Tronick, E.Z. and Field, T. (eds) (1986) *Maternal Depression and Infant Disturbance*, New Directions for Child Development, No. 34. San Francisco: Jossey Bass.

Tronick, E.Z. and Weinberg, M.K. (1997) 'Depressed Mothers and Infants: Failure to Form Dyadic States of Consciousness.' In L. Murray and P.J. Cooper (eds) *Postpartum Depression and Child Development*. New York: Guilford Press.

Vygotsky, L.S. (1967) 'Play and its role in the mental development of the child.' *Soviet Psychology 5*, 3, 6–18. Republished in J.S. Bruner, A. Jolly and K. Sylva (eds) (1985) *Play – Its Role in Development and Evolution*. Harmondsworth: Penguin.

Further reading

Bråten, S. (ed.) (2007) *On Being Moved: From Mirror Neurons to Empathy*. Amsterdam/Philadelphia: John Benjamins.

Bullowa, M. (ed.) (1979) *Before Speech: The Beginning of Human Communication*. London: Cambridge University Press.

Jaffe, J. and Felstein, S. (1970) *Rhythms of Dialogue*. New York: Academic Press.

Langer, S. (1953) *Feeling and Form: A Theory of Art Developed From Philosophy in a New Key*. London: Routledge and Kegan Paul.

Murray, L. and Andrews, L. (2000) *The Social Baby: Understanding Babies' Communication from Birth*. Richmond, Surrey: CP Publishing.

Murray, L. and Cooper, P.J. (eds) (1997) *Postpartum Depression and Child Development*. New York: Guilford Press.

Nadel, J. and Butterworth, G. (1999) (eds) *Imitation in Infancy*. Cambridge: Cambridge University Press.

Papoušek, H., Jürgens, U. and Papoušek, M. (1992) *Nonverbal Vocal Communication: Comparative and Developmental Aspects*. Cambridge: Cambridge University Press/Paris: Editions de la Maison des Sciences de l'Homme.

Reddy, V. and Trevarthen, C. (2004) 'What we learn about babies from engaging with their emotions.' *Zero to Three 24*, 3, 9–15.

Rizzolatti, G., Fogassi, L. and Gallese, V. (2006) 'Mirrors in the mind.' *Scientific American 295*, 5, 30–37.

Schore, A.N. (1994) *Affect Regulation and the Origin of the Self: The Neurobiology of Emotional Development*. Hillsdale, NJ: Erlbaum.

Stern, D.N. (2000) *The Interpersonal World of the Infant: A View from Psychoanalysis and Development Psychology*, 2nd edn, with new introduction. New York: Basic Books.

Thompson, E. (ed.) (2001) *Between Ourselves: Second-Person Issues in the Study of Consciousness*. Charlottesville, VA/Thorverton, UK: Imprint Academic. Also *Journal of Consciousness Studies 8*, 5–7.

Trainor, L.J. (2002) 'Lullabies and playsongs: Why we sing to children.' *Zero to Three 23*, 1, 31–34.

Trevarthen, C. (2005a) 'Action and Emotion in Development of the Human Self, its Sociability and Cultural Intelligence: Why Infants have Feelings like Ours.' In J. Nadel and D. Muir (eds) *Emotional Development*. Oxford: Oxford University Press.

Trevarthen, C. (2005b) 'Stepping away from the Mirror: Pride and Shame in Adventures of Companionship. Reflections on the Nature and Emotional Needs of Infant Intersubjectivity.' In C.S. Carter, L. Ahnert, K.E. Grossman, S.B. Hrdy, M.E. Lamb, S.W. Porges and N. Sachser (eds) *Attachment and Bonding: A New Synthesis*, Dahlem Workshop Report 92. Cambridge, MA: MIT Press.

Trevarthen, C. (2006) 'First things first: Infants make good use of the sympathetic rhythm of imitation, without reason or language.' *Journal of Child Psychotherapy 31*, 1, 91–113.

Trevarthen, C. and Aitken, K.J. (2001) 'Infant intersubjectivity: Research, theory, and clinical applications.' *Annual Research Review. The Journal of Child Psychology and Psychiatry and Allied Disciplines 42*, 1, 3–48.

Trevarthen, C., Aitken, K.J., Vandekerckhove, M., Delafield-Butt, J. and Nagy, E. (2006) 'Collaborative Regulations of Vitality in Early Childhood: Stress in Intimate Relationships and Postnatal Psychopathology.' In D. Cicchetti and D.J. Cohen (eds) *Developmental Psychopathology, Volume 2 Developmental Neuroscience*, 2nd edn. New York: Wiley.

Trevarthen, C. and Malloch, S. (2002) 'Musicality and music before three: Human vitality and invention shared with pride.' *Zero to Three 23*, 1, 10–18.

CHAPTER 3

THE UNIVERSALITY OF MUSICAL COMMUNICATION

Raymond A.R. MacDonald

We are all musical. Every human being has a biological, social and cultural guarantee of musicianship. Of course this is not a new idea and this observation has roots in educational and medical practice that date back to ancient Greek civilisation and probably beyond (Horden 2001). Neither is this notion a vague utopian ideal, but rather a conclusion drawn by an increasing number of academic researchers involved in investigating the foundations of musical behaviour. As Colwyn Trevarthen has shown in Chapter 2, the earliest communication between a parent and a child is essentially musical and, more specifically, improvisational. Indeed, to respond emotionally to music may be one defining feature of our humanity. Therefore music plays an absolutely fundamental communicative role in the earliest and most important relationship that we form in our lives, the relationship with our parents. In that sense we are all musical and we all have a musical identity because at that crucial point in our lives we were communicating musically and improvising with our parents.

In the following chapter I would like to unpack some of the implications of that opening statement: *we are all musical.* I will explore several themes. First of all, that we all have a musical identity. Second, that we all can and do use music for a variety of important communicative purposes. Finally, I will provide evidence to show how individuals with learning difficulties can learn musical skills, and will show how these music skills can be related to wider psychological developments and, in particular, communication.

It is important to note that I am writing this chapter from two different, yet related, perspectives. One is as psychologist, who specialises in researching the psychology of music from a variety of methodological and theoretical perspectives. The second is as a saxophonist who spends a considerable amount of time involved in improvising, with a particular interest in the communicative potential of spontaneous musical interactions. I have a firm belief that music is not only a separate, vital and hugely influential channel of communication, but that in the right context music can serve as a powerful therapeutic type of communication. Its use can also facilitate the development of wider, more general communication skills. I aim to convey this belief in the communicative potential of music through a number of theoretical, methodological and experimental examples in the following paragraphs.

We all have a musical identity

If you ask young people to describe themselves, they may tell you their age, they may tell you where they live, they may tell you what they study, but right at the top of that list they will tell you what music they like. They will use music as a badge of identity to signal to the world who they are. There is now quite compelling evidence to suggest that in terms of where young people socialise, the clothes they wear, the magazines they read, and the friendship groups that they socialise in, music plays an absolutely crucial role (MacDonald, Miell and Hargreaves 2002; Zillman and Gan 1997). In fact Zillman and Gan (1997) suggest that music is the most important recreational activity that young people are engaged in.

So music is a crucial aspect of a young person's identity. We are currently undertaking some work at Caledonian University investigating musical communication through the lifespan, exploring the extent to which music remains a crucial part of a person's identity in later life and also how musical identity develops and changes over the course of the lifespan. We organise focus groups and ask participants to talk about themselves. Quite quickly, music comes into the conversation. So in that sense as well, we are all musical. We all have a musical identity. What we are finding is that an older person's tastes certainly become broader and less affiliated to a particular genre of music, but we have clear evidence that music remains a key influence on people's identity. Music is still being used as a way of signalling to the world who the participants are.

Musical identities and communication

I have highlighted three of the possible ways of thinking about musical identity, but there are actually countless more ways of thinking of our musical identities. As well as music playing a crucial role in identities, it can also be viewed as a fundamental channel of communication, a channel separate from language. Music can facilitate the sharing of emotions, intentions and meanings, even though spoken language may be mutually incomprehensible (Miell, MacDonald and Hargreaves 2005). So, for example, if you are on a beach at Hogmanay with people from lots of different nationalities who may not speak English, they can all get together and sing some Beatles songs and unite through music. Not through the language but through the sense of unity that singing songs provides. We can communicate emotions, intentions and meanings through music (Cross 2005; Hodges 1996).

Also, music can provide a lifeline to human interaction for people who can't communicate through language for whatever reason. For such people, music can provide a fundamental lifeline to communication. The profession of music therapy now has 60 or 70 years of research looking at the processes and outcomes of music in a clinical setting and the way in which music can operate in these very particular clinical settings. There is extensive evidence of the powerful physical effects, and deep and profound emotional effects, that listening to and playing music can have (Magee 2002).

For example, Juslin and Sloboda (2001) document the vast number of ways in which music has a profound effect upon us emotionally. In this context I'm talking about music as a fundamental channel of communication. So not only does music play a crucial role in our identity construction and our negotiation of our identity, but music is also a fundamental channel of communication, playing a very important role in communicating emotions. Individuals who are involved in musical participation develop personal identities that are intrinsically musical.

By that I don't just mean professional musicians, such as an opera singer developing his or her musical identity as an opera singer. Regardless of your musical involvement, you have an identity as a musician. You might say 'I just sing in the bath' or 'I play a few Bob Dylan songs on the guitar', but once you are involved in any kind of musical activity you start to develop a sense of yourself as a musician. Another important point to note is that the identity of being a musician is a socially and culturally defined concept. It is not the case that an individual goes to university or college and attains a degree in music, secures a job as a musician and then adopts the label musician, the way in which medical doctors will go to university, study for many years, then, eventually, after practising and studying, they are allowed to call themselves a medical doctor. We don't acquire the label 'musician' after the attainment of advanced technical skills. It is not the case that we practise and practise and get better and better technically, and then suddenly confer the label 'musician' on ourselves. It has much more to do with the way in which our social and cultural surroundings are constructed and the way in which we relate to people around us (Borthwick and Davidson 2002).

For example, we have interviewed people with degrees in music who spend much of their life playing music but do not see themselves as a musician. They may say, for example, 'well actually my father was lead violin in a symphony orchestra, he is the musician in the family'. Although they have been playing music for 30 years, these individuals will not see themselves as musicians. So people with very advanced musical skills sometimes do not see themselves as musicians because there is someone else in their life who is 'better' than they are, or there are factors that lead them to reject adopting the label 'musician'. Thus the way in which the family is constructed has vital influence upon how we see ourselves as musicians.

On the other hand, we speak to 12-year-old children who don't have any formal education in music but have a band that practises in the garage every night. They consider themselves 'musicians'. That is their life; they are a musician now and they intend to remain a musician, so they have taken on the label 'musician'. The key point here is that we are talking about the notion of a musician as a socially constructed label and not something acquired after years of practice. There is also, as I have started to suggest here, the notion of being a musician as influenced by certain non-musical factors, what might be thought of as 'identity paradoxes' (MacDonald, Miell and Hargreaves 2002).

We have also interviewed jazz musicians, in order to investigate how their identity develops, how they see themselves and how they define jazz music. There are a huge number of ways in which a jazz musician is influenced by non-musical factors. Our findings show, for example, that jazz musicians see themselves as undervalued and not being paid appropriately enough for their concerts, and as being misunderstood. One of the defining features of being a jazz musician in the group we interviewed seemed to be that they felt people did not really understand what they were doing. They then used that as a way of sticking together and working together (MacDonald and Wilson 2005, 2006; Wilson and MacDonald 2005).

Sounds of Progress

The discussion above presents a brief overview of a number of theoretical issues relating to musical identities and musical communication, emphasising the importance that music has in our lives. They unpack, in a little bit more detail, this notion that we are all musical. What I would like to do now is to discuss a number of research projects that shed more light on this notion of us all being musical.

AIMS AND OBJECTIVES

These studies centre on my work with Sounds of Progress (SOP), a music production company based in Glasgow. They are an integrated music company who work with professional musicians and also with musicians and actors who have special needs. SOP work in hospitals and school settings, including running music workshops for developing basic music skills. SOP also work in special schools, carrying out recording and touring projects. There are a range of musical and social aims around the company. I started work with SOP as a musician working on gamelan workshops – in which participants form an orchestra comprised of bronze gongs, bells, and other 'metallophone' instruments. These instruments are easy and fun to learn to play, and thus make an excellent base for developing musical skills. Our efforts at this point were directed particularly toward facilitating such skills for individuals with mild to moderate learning difficulties. My own anecdotal observations of a group with whom I had worked for about six months was that they were making significant progress, and I found myself wondering if it was possible to gain an experimental view of what was happening at the workshops. So I decided to try to investigate the process and outcomes of this kind of intervention in a bit more detail.

METHODS

We investigated the process and outcomes of SOP's activities with 60 participants. All the participants were resident at the time in a large hospital. All participants had mild or moderate learning difficulties and there were 20 participants each in three groups:

1.   a group who participated in gamelan workshops once a week for three months

2.   an intervention control group, who were experiencing an intervention every week for three months that did *not* involve any music (i.e. cooking and art classes in the occupational therapy department)

3.   a non-intervention control group who did not take part in any special intervention relating to what we were doing here.

All participants in the groups were assessed before and after the sessions on musical ability, communication skills and self-perception of musical ability. Everyone was interviewed and assessed on their basic music skills, particularly rhythm and pitch. We also used a communication assessment profile used by speech therapists to quantify communication skills (Van der Gaag 1990). And we asked participants questions about their self-perceptions about their musical ability.

RESULTS

After the three months we found that in the experimental group there were significant improvements in musical ability. We were able to show statistically that the group of people coming to the gamelan workshop got better at playing music, in comparison to the other two groups who didn't have the intervention. Interestingly, their communication skills also developed. Using the Communication Assessment Profile for Adults with a Mental Handicap (CASP), we found a significant improvement in communication skills over the three months – improvements that were related to the music skills. The better participants got at music, the more their communication skills seemed to develop. There was also appreciable development in their self-perception of musical ability.

So these findings offer support, or examples, of the points that we are all musical, in the sense that we can all develop basic music skills, with the right type of intervention, and that music can have other effects on personal development. For this population, being involved in playing music not only improved music skills, but improved communication skills (MacDonald, Davies and O'Donnell 1999; O'Donnell, MacDonald and Davies 1999).

A QUALITATIVE STUDY

The project outlined above was an experimental study where we quantified the notion of musical ability into discrete variables such as rhythm and pitch, and we also focused on a very discrete measure of communication. It was clear to me that there was a lot more going on at the workshops than just these discrete variables. It was not just that the participants were developing rhythm awareness or their ability to label and talk about a photograph (which is what the CASP measures). We wanted to try to get some purchase on the wider developments that were being made and the meaning that music had in the lives of the people involved in SOP activities. So we utilised a qualitative research methodology. This particular study utilised the Social Model of Disability, which offers a social constructionist view of identity. It maintains that people's identity is constantly evolving, constantly being negotiated, and that all our experiences are very different and subjective. To get an understanding of an individual's personality therefore, we need to take a more subjective and holistic approach to studying personality (MacDonald and Miell 2002).

So we embarked on a qualitative study that included a number of structured interviews with participants who had all been involved in SOP activities for a number of years. These interviews were tape recorded and transcribed. Through repeated listening, we coded and refined the themes that emerged from these interviews. Rather than asking what *we* thought was important in music, we let the participants tell us what *they* thought.

The first theme that emerged related to how being involved in musical participation seemed to change the way in which other people viewed the participants, as illustrated in this quote:

> I remember I used to go up in the ambulance to the hospital years ago and there was this old woman who was always complaining about her illness. We used to call her 57 varieties. She always used to say about me, 'You know he's in a wee world of his own and you're sitting listening. You're sitting listening. Oh aye, I'm in a wee world of my own here.' Then again, that same old woman – I started a sing song in the ambulance one time she started to talk. And she started talking to me normally. You know what I mean? So there you go, she forgot about the 'world of my own' and when a sing song was started, she changed.

The key point here is that being involved in musical activities changes how other people view you. We saw this time and time again in the transcriptions. People talked about playing music, whether performing or recording, but when people started to play music, the outside world's view of that individual changed. That had a very strong effect on their self-concept and upon their sense of identity.

The second theme related to the importance of professionalism.

> When people spoke to you, they weren't giving you the sympathy vote any more. You know, I thought 'well I must be doing all right' you know. You didn't get all that 'pat on the head' and all that 'very good son'. Then you stop to think, 'well these disabled folk, what can they do?' Well I think they get rather a shock when they hear us. Then when things started to get a wee bit professional, I thought 'this can't be bad'.

As people develop their skill, we try to make sure that people get paid for their performances. This is the professional approach of SOP. If participants are going to record and go on tour, there is an expectation that participants are going to be performing and contributing in a professional manner, regardless of any learning difficulties they may have. SOP is giving people the chance to develop skills to a high standard. This aspect of our approach, this non-patronising way of working with people, seemed to have a very important effect on people's self-perceptions. They expected people to contribute significantly to the musical process, and when they were able to deliver it had a very powerful effect upon their sense of self.

The results from the experimental studies had highlighted the effects that music interventions can have on discrete personal and social factors. The analysis of the interview material suggested that involvement in musical activities also has more general effects on the way in which people think about themselves and about their position within society. These two developments are related in that music can be thought of as not only facilitating specific changes in musical and psychological factors, but also as contributing to the identity projects in which the individuals are engaged. Whilst we have been focusing our discussion upon the activities of one particular music company, SOP, our team intends it as an example of how *any* musical participation, suitably structured, can be an excellent vehicle for achieving musical and personal communicative gains for participants – including individuals with 'special needs' (Mac-

Donald, Miell and Wilson 2005). These effects will not be found only in participants in SOP. When music is employed for therapeutic/educational objectives in a structured and goal-directed way, by individuals with musical expertise and training, then outcomes of the type reported here can be expected (Pavlicevic and Ansdell 2004).

Summary

I have looked at musical identities, I have given a broad overview of some issues relating to musical identities and musical communication and I have talked about music in special education and special needs. Music is not a magic bullet or the ultimate panacea. I am not trying to suggest that just by playing music we change our lives or just by listening to music it is going to help with all personal challenges. Rather, music needs to be utilised in a knowledgeable way and, when that is done, it can have very significant effects. I hope that the work I have described illustrates the wide range of domains on which music can have such effects. Unfortunately, Western society constructs an elitist image of musicians, and this has negative implications for us all – all of us who feel 'I am not musical so I am not able to play music,' disabled and non-disabled alike. The work that we are doing seeks to change the unhelpful way in which society currently constructs it notion of 'musician'.

References

Borthwick, S.J. and Davidson, J.W. (2002) 'Personal Identity and Music: A Family Perspective.' In R.A.R. MacDonald, D.J. Hargreaves and D. Miell (eds) *Musical Identities.* Oxford: Oxford University Press.

Cross, I. (2005) 'Music and Meaning, Ambiguity and Evolution.' In D. Miell, R.A.R. MacDonald and D.J. Hargreaves (eds) *Musical Communication.* Oxford: Oxford University Press.

Hodges, D.A. (eds) (1996) *Handbook of Music Psychology.* San Antonio, TX: IMR Press.

Horden, P. (ed.) (2001) *Music as Medicine.* Aldershot: Ashgate Publishing.

Juslin, P.N. and Sloboda, J.A. (eds) (2001) *Music and Emotion.* Oxford: Oxford University Press.

MacDonald, R.A.R., Davies, J.B. and O'Donnell, P.J. (1999) 'Structured music workshops for individuals with learning difficulty: An empirical investigation.' *Journal of Applied Research in Intellectual Disabilities 12*, 3, 225–241.

MacDonald, R.A.R. and Miell, D. (2002) 'Music for Individuals with Special Needs: A Catalyst for Developments in Identity, Communication and Musical Ability.' In R.A.R. Mac-

Donald, D.J. Hargreaves and D. Miell (eds) *Musical Identities*. Oxford: Oxford University Press.

MacDonald, R.A.R., Hargreaves, D.J. and Miell, D. (eds) (2002) *Musical Identities*. Oxford: Oxford University Press.

MacDonald, R.A.R., Miell, D. and Wilson, G.B. (2005) 'Talking about Music: A Vehicle for Identity Development.' In D. Miell, R.A.R. MacDonald and D.J. Hargreaves (eds) *Musical Communication*. Oxford: Oxford University Press.

MacDonald, R.A.R. and Wilson, G.B. (2005) 'The musical identities of professional jazz musicians: A focus group investigation.' *Psychology of Music 33*, 4, 395–419.

MacDonald, R.A.R. and Wilson, G.B. (2006) 'Constructions of jazz: How jazz musicians present their collaborative musical practice.' *Musicae Scientiae 10*, 1, 59–85.

Magee, W.L. (2002) 'Disability and Identity in Music Therapy.' In R.A.R. MacDonald, D.J. Hargreaves and D. Miell (eds) *Musical Identities*. Oxford: Oxford University Press.

Miell, D., MacDonald, R.A.R and Hargreaves, D.J. (eds) (2005) *Musical Communication*. Oxford: Oxford University Press.

O'Donnell, P.J., MacDonald, R.A.R. and Davies, J.B. (1999) 'Video Analysis of the Effects of Structured Music Workshops for Individuals with Learning Difficulties.' In D. Erdonmez and R.R. Pratt (eds) *Music Therapy and Music Medicine: Expanding Horizons*. Saint Louis, MO: MMB Music.

Pavlicevic, M. and Ansdell, G. (2004) *Community Music Therapy*. London: Jessica Kingsley Publishers.

Van der Gaag, A. (1990) 'The validation of a language and communication assessment procedure for use with adults with intellectual disabilities.' *Health Bulletin 48*, 5, 254–260.

Wilson, G.B. and MacDonald, R.A.R. (2005) 'The meaning of the blues: Musical identities in talk about jazz.' *Qualitative Research in Psychology 2*, 341–363.

Zillman, D. and Gan, S. (1997) 'Musical Taste in Adolescence.' In D.J. Hargreaves and A.C. North (eds) *The Social Psychology of Music*. London: Oxford University Press.

PART 2

Communicative Impairments

CHAPTER 4

THE USE OF IMITATION WITH CHILDREN WITH AUTISTIC SPECTRUM DISORDER: FOUNDATIONS FOR SHARED COMMUNICATION

Michelle B. O'Neill, Martyn C. Jones and M. Suzanne Zeedyk

'my sense of myself grows by my imitation of you and my sense of yourself grows in terms of myself'

James Mark Baldwin (1897/1995, p.9)

Baldwin put the topic of imitation on the 'psychological map' more than a century ago. Much investigation of this phenomenon has since been carried out, and one of the many insights it has generated is the growing evidence that using imitation with children with Autistic Spectrum Disorder (ASD) nurtures their communicative abilities. When adults imitate the behaviours of children with ASD, the children become more socially engaged: smiling, looking more often at the adult, initiating more elements of the interaction and taking more turns in an exchange. It would appear that when the adult joins the world of the child, by using the child's behaviours and interests, the child is presented with an inherently interesting and recognisable 'language'. A crucial starting point for effective interaction has been created.

The aim of this chapter is to describe this process in more detail, showing how the use of imitation with children with ASD can increase communicative and social behaviours. The chapter starts with an overview of ASD before moving on to a review of recent work on the use of imitation with children with ASD. One of the studies from our own research (O'Neill 2007; submitted by the first author for the degree of PhD and supervised by the co-authors of this paper) on the use of imitation by parents/carers with children with ASD is also described, showing in particular the changes in behaviour that occur when imitation is introduced into play interactions. The chapter ends with an exploration of why imitation is so effective and what this outcome tells us about shared and meaningful communication. All of these issues have important consequences for how we come to understand and engage in communication, regardless of our particular communicative styles and preferences.

An overview of Autistic Spectrum Disorder

Autistic Spectrum Disorder is categorised in the International Classification of Diseases 10 (ICD-10 2006) under three main labels: Childhood Autism (also known as Classical Autism), Atypical Autism and Asperger's Syndrome. Each of these is defined according to age of onset and behavioural manifestations. Childhood Autism, for example, appears before three years of age and consists of impairments in the development of reciprocal social interaction and communication, and restricted, stereotyped, repetitive behaviour. These three areas of development are also referred to as the 'triad of impairments'. In addition to difficulties in these areas, other problems such as phobias, sleeping and eating disturbances, temper tantrums and self-directed aggression may also be present (ICD-10 2006).

In terms of social interaction, an individual with ASD may find it difficult to relate to others, may have problems with interpersonal development, can find social cues and signals problematic and anxiety-provoking (due to them being hard to understand) and can sometimes appear to be detached from others. Language and communication can be problematic, with language acquisition being delayed or difficulty being experienced in understanding the subtleties associated with linguistic acts such as sarcasm and analogy. Thought and behavioural difficulties may also occur in relation to activities such as pretend and imaginative play. As one of the main features of ASD is rigidity of thought, participating in activities that require abstract and flexible thought can be problematic. Moreover, behaviour can become ritualised, obsessive and exclusive, and both unexpected and planned changes to routine can cause distress (Frith 2003;

Happé 1994; Public Health Institute of Scotland 2001; Trevarthen *et al.* 1999; Wing 1996).

Although the number of cases of ASD in children and adults appears to be increasing, reports on the actual prevalence of autism differ from source to source. Authors (e.g. Prior 2003; Prior *et al.* 1998; Volkmar *et al.* 2004; Wing 1993; Wing and Potter 2002) have pointed out that several factors may contribute to changes in rates of ASD: the diagnostic system used, interpretations of the diagnostic system, the sampling methods used in describing traits and manifestations, the type and methodology of the studies carried out, and actual increases in the number of individuals with ASD. Nonetheless, the rate of prevalence is undeniably worrying, with a recent publication suggesting that the rates of ASD in children may be as high as 1 in 100 children (Baird *et al.* 2006).

Creating meaningful interactions: Approaches that facilitate shared communication through shared language

Many approaches have been developed specifically for individuals with ASD to support communication and social interactions. One particular type of approach involves the use of an individual's own actions and gestures, facial expressions, interest and motivations in everyday communication. This approach can be seen in the use of Intensive Interaction with individuals with multiple and complex needs (e.g. Caldwell 2006; Ephraim 1979; Nind and Hewett 2001) and the use of imitation with children with ASD in research studies (e.g. Heimann, Laberg and Nordøen 2006; Nadel and Pezé 1993; Nadel *et al.* 2000).

INTENSIVE INTERACTION

Intensive Interaction involves the observation of an individual's behaviours and the use of elements of those behaviours to establish communication. Behaviours that could be meaningful include actions, gestures, vocalisations (e.g. words, noises, singing, whistling), repetitive behaviours and self-stimulatory behaviours. Once the behaviours have been noted, a communicative partner can use them to open up a dialogue with the person with ASD, as Coia and Jardine Handley describe in more detail in Chapter 7. For example, if an individual enjoys tapping repetitively on the wall humming a tune, the other person might tap on the door in the same rhythm, also humming the tune. Care must be taken to gauge the individual's response to this, and knowledge of the individual and his or her likes and dislikes is important in ensuring the feeling of wellbeing and safety in the individual (e.g. hypersensitivities, preferences for personal space, susceptibility to feeling overwhelmed).

Of particular interest is the work of Phoebe Caldwell, who has used the approach for several decades as a practitioner, and has specialised in the use of Intensive Interaction with people with ASD. As she has described in her numerous publications (e.g. Caldwell 2003, 2006), including Chapter 11 in this volume, Caldwell uses Intensive Interaction to reduce the 'sensory chaos' and stress experienced by some individuals with ASD and thus to establish communication. Drawing on the work of Ephraim (1979) and Nind and Hewett (2001), Caldwell refers to Intensive Interaction as 'learning the language' of an individual. The conceptualisation of an individual's behaviour as his or her 'language' is crucial in our understanding of his or her sensory, social and personal world. Indeed, conceiving of behaviour in this way is fundamental to the development of a mutually communicative relationship. In this respect, all behaviour, no matter how small or subtle, can be considered as part of an individual's language.

THE USE OF IMITATION WITH CHILDREN WITH ASD

Imitation has been used in other therapeutic programmes and has been shown to be effective in encouraging sociability and interactivity in children with ASD. There is considerable overlap in these programmes with the approach of Intensive Interaction, but it is notable that some practitioners of Intensive Interaction resist the term 'imitation' because it carries the connotation of only mirroring the partner, rather than *responding* to the partner in his or her own language. Many of the researchers who use the term 'imitation' are comfortable with it because they have moved into the study of this area after working initially in the area of infant communication (as described in Chapter 2), and ultimately see themselves as pursuing the same aim as Intensive Interaction: encouraging communication and meaningful social interaction. The importance of terminology is a debate that probably deserves more attention in the literature: what are the consequences, for our understanding of the processes involved, of using or of avoiding the term 'imitation'?

When imitation and Intensive Interaction are discussed, they are sometimes termed 'interventions', as is illustrated throughout this book.

This is a misnomer in some ways, for Intensive Interaction and imitation are better viewed as a style of communication, to be used consistently rather than for set periods of time deemed as 'intervention sessions'. There is, however, value in conceiving of this approach as an intervention within the research context, for this provides a framework for systematically measuring the effect of these approaches – information that is crucial for building up evidence-based practice. Without a reliable evidence base it is difficult to identify precisely which aspects of an approach are most effective and, therefore, how the approach can be further developed and applied on a large scale.

Early studies showed that adult imitations of the behaviour of children with ASD result in the duration and frequency of children's eye gaze increasing (Dawson and Adams 1984; Tiegerman and Primavera 1984). Dawson and Adams (1984) also showed that the experimenter's imitation of the child resulted in more socially responsive behaviour and less pervasive play. Harris, Handleman and Fong (1987) found that when an adult imitated the self-stimulatory behaviour of children with ASD the children's levels of happiness increased. Dawson and Galpert (1990) showed that children with ASD gazed at their mother's face more and engaged more in creative toy play when imitated by their mother. Likewise, children with ASD were found to be more socially engaged with the experimenter in an imitative play condition (Lewy and Dawson 1992).

Over the past two decades Jacqueline Nadel, based in France, has carried out leading work in this area. Some of her initial work, conducted with colleagues (Nadel and Pezé 1993), reported on her efforts working with a 10-year-old boy with ASD, over a period of a year. Duplicate sets of toys were provided, in order that synchronous imitation could take place. One of the pair would spend hour-long sessions with the child, using imitation and encouraging the child to imitate in return. The findings showed that over the course of the year, there were noticeable increases in the social gestures, physical contact and laughter and smiling of the child. The boy also spent less time imitating and more time engaging in and initiating more cooperative and complementary exchanges, suggesting that imitation 'can serve as a template for other forms of exchanges' (Nadel and Pezé 1993, p.150). Thus, as with the outcomes from practitioners, research evidence suggests that imitation not only encourages communicative exchanges, it also fosters the development of the communicative relationship between two individuals, allowing them to move from imitation into other communicative exchanges. The 'conversation' can progress and develop.

In a later study Nadel *et al.* (2000) employed what is known as the 'still face paradigm' to test the expectations of children with ASD regarding the behaviours of unfamiliar people. They used three three-minute sessions that took place in the following order:

1. The adult adopted a statue-like appearance with a still face and body (still face 1).

2. The adult imitated the behaviours of the child (imitation interaction session).

3. The adult returned to still face behaviour (still face 2).

It was found that in the first session, the children seemed not to notice the adult, spending little time looking at him or her, showing any emotional expressions, touching the adult, or displaying any social gestures. None of the children appeared to be distressed or concerned about the adult's still face behaviour.

In the second session, where the adult imitated the child, there were significant changes in the children's behaviour: they looked at the adult, touched him or her and used more positive social gestures. These shifts indicated that they were becoming more involved in communicating with the adult. It seemed remarkable that such changes could be achieved in the brief space of only three minutes.

In the final session (still face 2), the adult returned to statue-like behaviour. The children's response was striking. They looking away much more often, and displayed negative facial expressions. Their positive social gestures and emotional expressions decreased substantially. This change is so notable because, in the first still face condition, the children had showed no interest in the experimenter and had made no effort to initiate interaction. In this final session, however, the children were uncomfortable with, even disturbed by, the adult's use of statue-like behaviour. Imitation had created an expectation that the adult would respond socially and sensitively to the child – and therefore disappointment when the adult was inactive.

Nadel *et al.* suggest that imitation allows the children to see themselves as like the imitating adult, which should result in the children viewing 'others as human beings like themselves' (Nadel *et al.* 2000, p.135). This encourages the development of social expectations, causing the children to appear 'to react to a social rule violation only after the adult had been recognised as a human being' (p.143). That is, the use of imitation results in the child experiencing, and therefore recognising, the social nature of the adult's behaviour.

Nadel's work has now been replicated by other research teams using designs similar to the one she developed (Escalona *et al.* 2002; Field *et al.* 2001; Heimann *et al.* 2006). The results of this work all support the finding that imitation is effective in establishing communicative interactions and social expectancies amongst children with ASD. Moreover, work conducted by other teams, such as those led by Ingersoll (e.g. Ingersoll and Schreibman 2006) and Greenspan and Wieder (1999; Greenspan, Wieder and Simons 1998), are producing similar results, while using very different designs. Overall, it is becoming apparent that children with ASD do have a desire to interact and play creatively with other people. Imitation seems to be able to play a key role in unlocking this ability within them.

A study on parents'/carers' use of imitation as an intervention

In our own research programme we have set out to apply these insights in a new way. We have been exploring the extent to which parents and carers can make use of an imitative style of interacting with their child with ASD. As part of the first author's PhD thesis, a study was carried out to test the effectiveness of imitation as an intervention used by parent or carers. Based on the work of Nadel and her colleagues, we predicted that increasing parents'/carers' imitations of their child would result in increases in the child's social behaviours. Four dyads of parents/carers and their child took part in the study. We had two main elements to the study: introducing duplicate toys into play, because this encourages spontaneous imitation, and providing training to parents in the use of imitation. Thus the study asked two main questions:

1. To what extent does the use of a duplicate set of toys succeed in promoting spontaneous imitation between parents and children with ASD?

2. Is a short training session in using imitation effective in increasing the amount of imitation shown by parents/carers and, if so, what are the effects of this increased imitation on the child's behaviours?

To answer the first question, each adult and child took part in several play sessions, all of which were filmed with the adult's written permission. A total of six sessions, over the period of a few visits, took place. In the first few sessions they were invited to play with a selection of toys that we provided (such as balloons, children's umbrellas, cymbals, hats, large plastic toy springs) in whichever way they wanted. This was meant to provide a baseline measure of 'standard play', so only one set of each toy was provided, as it is common to find only single sets of toys in most houses and play situations. Over the next few sessions though, the parent and child were provided with duplicate sets of toys (e.g. two balloons, two children's umbrellas, two sets of cymbals), as Nadel had done in her research studies. We videotaped these sessions and later analysed the actions of adults and children using sophisticated microanalytic coding techniques, which allowed us to look in detail at selected behaviours.

Of particular interest in this study was parent imitation (how often the parent imitated the child), turn taking (how many turns were taken within the exchanges between the dyad), child initiation of play (how often the child directed the play that was occurring). The analysis of the play sessions showed that when the single-toy sessions were compared with the duplicate-toy sessions, there were improvements on all fronts between the first and last sessions. Parents' spontaneous imitation of the children typically doubled ($p<.02$); turn taking within the session tended to increase by three instances or more ($p<.03$), and the children's initiation of activities increased by half or more, showing that they were taking more charge of the play that was happening ($p<.04$).

To answer the second question – is training effective in increasing parent imitation, and does this then give rise to increases in the child's social behaviours? – was explored by asking the dyads to take part in six more play sessions. In the first few of these sessions each pair were invited to play with the duplicate set of toys as they wished. The parent then took part in a short training session whereby the use of imitation was described and video footage of the author imitating a child, as well as footage of a child with ASD being imitated by the parent, was shown. (Prior written consent had been obtained in relation to showing the video footage.) The parent was free to ask questions throughout the training session.

Prior to the next play session, the parent was reminded of the discussion in the training session and was then asked to imitate the child as much as possible in the upcoming play sessions. The results obtained from analysing the video footage confirmed that the training was effective: between the first and last of these sessions, parents' imitation of the children had increased by at least four instances (p<.02). This shift in behaviour had the desired impact on the overall interaction, with both turn taking (p<.03) and children's initiation of activities (p<.04) tending to double by the end of the sessions (p<.03). These results indicate that parents can use imitation in an intentional way and that, when they do, their children become more sociable, engaged and communicative.

Overall, we were very pleased with these outcomes. They show that intervening positively in the lives of families who have a child with ASD is neither time-consuming nor expensive. Simply introducing duplicate sets of toys changes the way that parents and children play, and providing even brief training sessions encouraging imitation can make a significant improvement in interactions. These findings offer considerable hope to families with children with ASD, as well as to social, education and health services seeking interventions that involve parents and carers.

Why is imitation so effective – what's happening?

The question of why imitation is so effective is a very interesting one. It could be discussed at length, not only in relation to ASD, but to other domains, such as infancy, learning disabilities, sensory impairment and dementia, as other chapters in this book amply illustrate. In this chapter our aim has been to focus on findings relating to the use of imitation with children with ASD, in the hope that this will whet the appetite of those wishing to explore its use further. We will conclude the chapter by summarising some of the explanations that have been provided by other authors as to why imitation seems to be so effective in promoting communication for children and adults with ASD. Although each of these explanations places a different emphasis on why imitation is effective, taken together they accord well in their accounts of why imitation has the kinds of effects that have been described in this chapter.

THE USE OF AN INDIVIDUAL'S LANGUAGE PROVIDES A GATEWAY TO ENGAGEMENT

Caldwell (2006) suggests that the use of an individual's own language (e.g. actions, gestures, vocalisations, topics of interest) provides a gateway to communication. Joining in another person's behaviours both reduces stress and acts as a personal code that both partners recognise and share in. Basing interactions on individuals' own behaviours creates a safe and recognisable language for communication – because it is their own language. The familiarity of that language induces interest, and makes it safe enough to move away from self-stimulating behaviours into shared interaction with another person. As Caldwell (2006, p.277) describes it, 'because the brain recognises its own signals, using Intensive Interaction shifts the focus of a person's attention from their locked-in inner world to the world outside'. Thus, the use of the individual's language provides a mutual base from which the two partners can develop a trustworthy, engaging relationship.

IMITATION CREATES SOCIAL EXPECTANCY AND A SENSE OF AGENCY

Nadel, Prepin and Okanda (2005) suggest that the increase in social awareness observed when children with ASD are imitated may arise as a result of their discovery of self-agency. They suggest that as the child produces a particular behaviour, he or she becomes aware of it taking place in another person (i.e. externally). This creates awareness that the child is not only the producer of his or her own act; the child is also the basis of the other person's act. As the imitative act occurs, the child becomes aware that he or she has a type of influence over the other person. In addition, the partner's imitations of the child set up an expectation in the child that the other person will engage with him or her. This is the reason that in the Nadel *et al.* (2000) study the children responded negatively to the second still face session: 'They understand the still behaviour as being at will. They now react to the still face like people typically react to ostracism…it is an insult to their being there' (Nadel *et al.* 2005, p.457). The adult's imitation creates social awareness and social expectation in the child, and, as such, the child reacts negatively when these expectations are not met (i.e. when the adult adopts a statue-like appearance). It is as though the adult's imitation of the child's behaviour has awakened the child's awareness of the communicative power of both him- or herself and the adult.

IMITATION PROVIDES THE CLOSEST EQUIVALENCE OF SELF AND OTHER

Zeedyk (2006) identifies imitation as one of many forms of communicative exchange. She argues, however, that it offers the closest equivalence of self and other, and that this quality gives it particular power as a means of communication. Zeedyk's view is that imitation creates emotional intimacy between two people, and as the communicating partners negotiate the behaviours to be shared, they learn about the boundaries of the interaction (how far can the boundaries be pushed, the emotions of the others played with, the shared components recognised even when taking a new form). Consequently, the pair learn about boundaries between self and other. Zeedyk (2006, p.332) describes this process as the 'essence of intersubjective engagement' and suggests that through these interactions, we come to learn about self. She also suggests that other capacities, such as self-awareness and representation, develop as a result of emotional intimacy with another human being. Thus, for Zeedyk, a fundamental means through which people learn about themselves, others and the world around them is through the emotional intimacy established during imitation.

IMITATION INCORPORATES THE KEY TENETS OF EFFECTIVE COMMUNICATION

Intensive Interaction and imitation encompass some of the essential ingredients required for effective, shared and meaningful communication. The use of imitation is powerful not only because of the impact it has on communication, but also because it informs us about the essence of what it is to communicate, regardless of one's neurological or developmental status. The principles underlying this approach, even for those who have not expressly voiced it this way, appear to be founded on valuing another person's humanity – that person's experience of his or her social and sensory world. We would agree; this attitude lies at the heart of all respectful interactions. The very act of observing and joining in with another person's behaviours encourages us to 'step back' and reduce the speed of our communication, thus creating space for the shared (and perhaps unpredicted) communicative response to emerge. The creation of this 'space' and change in pace may be particularly crucial for individuals with ASD, who often require extra time to process the flow of incoming information. As the communicative relationship progresses and develops between two people, the communicative repertoire can expand, with new topics of interest and new behaviours introduced by both partners. This allows both partners to share equally and removes the need for one partner to take the lead. In essence, the use of a *shared* language removes barriers and power struggles, creating a safe and recognisable domain within which people can engage with one another. When a common ground is reached, 'real' communication begins to take place. In this sense, imitation can be considered as laying down the stepping stones to a meeting place.

How can I use imitation with my child with ASD?

Some of the key resources for using approaches such as imitation and Intensive Interaction have already been cited in this chapter. Of particular relevance are texts by Nind and Hewett (e.g. 2001) and those by Caldwell (e.g. 2003, 2006). They give practical guidance and real-life examples on how Intensive Interaction can be used as an approach to communication. This earlier work is of course supplemented by other chapters in this volume.

The essence of an imitative approach is the inherent interest and valuing of the other persons' social, sensory and communicative world. In this sense, the building of a relationship through effective communication should incorporate genuine interest in the other person, observation and openness to what communication might mean to him or her – a willingness to adapt our own perceptions of communication to fit more harmoniously with our partner's. Imitation should form part of an approach which encompasses these elements, at the root of which should be the aim of genuinely shared interaction.

Our hope is that parents will become more aware of this approach, not only through reading material such as this, but also through being made aware of it by professionals. It would be easy for social, educational and health professionals to incorporate this way of working into advice that they give to parents. But first professionals must be provided with information and evidence of this approach. We are currently planning studies that would encourage such a shift: what actions need to happen within existing professional services to make staff aware of the outcomes we have been discussing here, and what kind of support do parents benefit from in attempting to embed it in their lives with their children with ASD?

Conclusion

Imitation clearly has the potential to be of use in engaging with children with ASD – whether for professionals, parents or carers. The power of imitation as an intervention approach lies in its underlying aim: to awaken and realise the communicative potential between two people, through the sharing of an individual's own language and interests. The principles of genuine interest in and care for another person's experience of the world lie at the core of all harmonious social interactions. They constitute the very basis of what it means to relate meaningfully as human beings. This, it can be argued, constitutes a key explanation as to why imitation and Intensive Interaction has been shown to be powerful not only for individuals with ASD but for so many other kinds of communicative difficulties. Recognising 'ourself in another' captures interest on many levels and provides the common ground for shared interaction. This is the basis for engaging with other people, regardless of the nature of their linguistic ability, in emotionally meaningful ways.

Acknowledgements

We would like to thank the children and parents/carers who participated in the study, and the preschool centre staff for their support and cooperation. The doctoral research described here was undertaken at the University of Dundee in part fulfilment of the first author's PhD degree, under the supervision of Dr Martyn C. Jones (School of Nursing and Midwifery) and Dr M. Suzanne Zeedyk (School of Psychology). Permission to carry out the study was granted by the Local Authority Education Department on 3 December 2003 and ethical approval was granted by the School of Psychology Ethics Committee, University of Dundee on 18 December 2003.

References

Baird, G., Simonoff, E., Pickles, A., Chandler, S., Loucas, T., Meldrum, D. and Charman, T. (2006) 'Prevalence of disorders of the autism spectrum in a population cohort of children in South Thames: The Special Needs and Autism Project (SNAP).' *Lancet 368*, 179–181.

Baldwin, J.M. (1897/1995) *Social and Ethical Interpretations in Mental Development: A Study in Social Psychology*. London: Routledge.

Caldwell, P. (2003) *Crossing the Minefield: Establishing Safe Passage through the Sensory Chaos of Autistic Spectrum Disorder*. Brighton: Pavilion Publishing.

Caldwell, P. (2006) *Finding You Finding Me: Using Intensive Interaction to Get in Touch with People whose Severe Learning Disabilities are Combined with Autistic Spectrum Disorder*. London: Jessica Kingsley Publishers.

Dawson, G. and Adams, A. (1984) 'Imitation and social responsiveness in autistic children.' *Journal of Abnormal Child Psychology 12*, 209–226.

Dawson, G. and Galpert, L. (1990) 'Mothers' uses of imitative play for facilitating social responsiveness and toy play in young autistic children.' *Development and Psychopathology 2*, 151–162.

Ephraim, G. (1979) 'Augmented mothering.' Unpublished paper. Bryn-y-Neuadd Hospital, Llanfairfechan, Gwynedd, North Wales.

Escalona, A., Field, T., Nadel, J. and Lundy, B. (2002) 'Brief report: Imitation effects on children with autism.' *Journal of Autism and Developmental Disorders 32*, 141–144.

Field, T., Field, T., Sanders, C., and Nadel, J. (2001) 'Children with autism display more social behaviors after repeated imitation sessions.' *Autism 5*, 3, 317–323.

Frith, U. (2003) *Autism: Explaining the Enigma.* Oxford: Blackwell.

Greenspan, S.I. and Wieder, S. (1999) 'A functional developmental approach to Autism Spectrum Disorders.' *Journal for the Association for Persons with Severe Handicaps 24*, 147–161.

Greenspan, S.I., Wieder, S. and Simons, R. (1998) *The Child with Special Needs: Encouraging Intellectual and Emotional Growth.* Jackson, TN: Perseus Books.

Happé, F. (1994) *Autism: An Introduction to Psychological Theory.* Hove: Psychology Press.

Harris, S.L., Handleman, J.S. and Fong, P.L. (1987) 'Imitation of self-stimulation: Impact on the autistic child's behavior and affect.' *Child and Family Behavior Therapy 9*, 1–21.

Heimann, M., Laberg, K.E. and Nordøen, B. (2006) 'Imitative interaction increases social interest and elicited imitation in non-verbal children with autism.' *Infant and Child Development 15*, 297–309.

ICD-10 (International Statistical Classification of Diseases and Related Health Problems 10) (2006) *Classification of Mental and Behavioural Disorders: Clinical Description and Diagnostic Guidelines.* Geneva: World Health Organization.

Ingersoll, B. and Schreibman, L. (2006) 'Teaching reciprocal imitation skills to young children with autism using a naturalistic behavioral approach: Effects on language, pretend play, and joint attention.' *Journal of Autism and Developmental Disorders 36*, 487–505.

Lewy, A.L. and Dawson, G. (1992) 'Social stimulation and joint attention in young autistic children.' *Journal of Abnormal Child Psychology 20*, 555–566.

Nadel, J., Croué, S., Mattlinger, M.-J., Canet, P., Hudelot, C., Lecuyer, C. and Martini, M. (2000) 'Do children with autism have expectancies about the social behaviour of unfamiliar people?' *Autism 4*, 133–145.

Nadel, J. and Pezé, A. (1993) 'What Makes Immediate Imitation Communicative in Toddlers and Autistic Children?' In J. Nadel and L. Camaioni (eds) *New Perspectives in Early Communicative Development.* London: Routledge.

Nadel, J., Prepin, K. and Okanda, M. (2005) 'Experiencing contingency and agency: First step toward self-understanding in making a mind?' *Interaction Studies 6*, 447–462.

Nind, M. and Hewett, D. (2001) *A Practical Guide to Intensive Interaction.* Plymouth, UK: BILD.

O'Neill, M.B. (2007) 'Imitation as an intervention for children with Autistic Spectrum Disorder and their parents/carers.' PhD thesis, University of Dundee.

Prior, M. (2003) 'Is there an increase in the prevalence of autism spectrum disorders?' *Journal of Paediatrics and Child Health 39*, 81–82.

Prior, M., Eisenmajer, R., Leekham, S., Wing, L., Gould, J., Ong, B. and Dowe, D. (1998) 'Are there subgroups within the autistic spectrum? A cluster analysis of a group of children with autistic spectrum disorders.' *Journal of Child Psychology and Psychiatry 39*, 893–902.

Public Health Institute of Scotland (2001, December) *Needs Assessment Report: Autistic Spectrum Disorders*. Glasgow, Scotland: Public Health Institute of Scotland, NHS Scotland.

Tiegerman, E. and Primavera, L.H. (1984) 'Imitating the autistic child: Facilitating communicative gaze behavior.' *Journal of Autism and Developmental Disorders 14*, 27–38.

Trevarthen, C., Aitken, K., Papoudi, D. and Robarts, J. (1999) *Children with Autism: Diagnosis and Interventions to Meet their Needs*. London: Jessica Kingsley Publishers.

Volkmar, F.R., Lord, C., Bailey, A., Schultz, R.T. and Klin, A. (2004) 'Autism and pervasive developmental disorders.' *Journal of Child Psychology and Psychiatry 45*, 135–170.

Wing, L. (1993) 'The definition and prevalence of autism: A review.' *European Child and Adolescent Psychiatry 2*, 61–74.

Wing, L. (1996) *The Autistic Spectrum*. London: Constable.

Wing, L. and Potter, D. (2002) 'The epidemiology of autistic spectrum disorders: Is the prevalence rising?' *Mental Retardation and Developmental Disabilities Research Reviews 8*, 151–161.

Zeedyk, M.S. (2006) 'From intersubjectivity to subjectivity: The transformative roles of emotional intimacy and imitation.' *Infant and Child Development 15*, 321–344.

CHAPTER 5

SHARING COMMUNICATIVE LANDSCAPES WITH CONGENITALLY DEAFBLIND PEOPLE: IT'S A WALK IN THE PARK!

Paul Hart

This chapter will suggest there is no theoretical reason why congenitally deafblind people should not be able to communicate using language. This view may strike some readers, including practitioners in the deafblind field, as surprising, but it is one that I have come to hold as a consequence of 20 years of practice, working alongside congenitally deafblind people. In this period I have seen countless communication breakdowns between congenitally deafblind people and their communication partners. I do not take this as an indication that language is an impossible goal, as some observers have done. Instead, I would argue that these breakdowns serve to highlight the attitudes and approaches that need to be adopted by communication partners if we are to understand the world of a congenitally deafblind person. I believe that, in this field, we can and should be moving towards 'shared communicative landscapes'.

Sacks (1995) suggested that 'when we open our eyes each morning, it is upon a world we have spent a lifetime learning to see' (p.108). Congenitally deafblind people have this experience as well – except that they do so by stretching out their hands each morning, upon a world that they have spent a lifetime learning to feel. Each of us has a different reality of the world, a world that we have been constructing since we were born and a world that mirrors the ways in which it has been perceived. For a congenitally deafblind person, whose pre-eminent source of contact with the outside world is through touch, we need to explore not so much what these 'shared communicative landscapes' look like but instead what they feel like, since the tactile modality is of primary importance for this group of people.

From a common touchpoint on the world, congenitally deafblind people and their communication partners can travel together on journeys where 'new worlds beckon' (Zeedyk 2006, p.330), journeys that ultimately allow them to draw on one of language's most important functions: being able to make reference to displaced objects and events that are not present at that time (Goldin-Meadow 2005). Reddy (2003) describes these as 'things external in space…[and] events distant in time' (p.398). Such journeys, however, must start from a secure 'companion space' (Kugiumutzakis 1998, p.63), where trust and respect for each other's perspective on the world is paramount. Nevertheless, it is primarily the responsibility of communication partners to think themselves into the perceptual world of the deafblind person and to participate in joint activities from that person's perspective. Language for congenitally deafblind people is likely to emerge from such joint activities and is likely to be based around the movements, gestures and actions that are used within the activity (Daelman *et al.* 1996, 1999b; Gibson 2005; Nafstad and Rødbroe 1999).

In exploring these topics, I will pose three questions in this chapter:

1. Is it theoretically possible for congenitally deafblind people to develop language?

2. What are the key features underpinning attitudes and approaches of communication partners?

3. What would an intervention designed to develop these 'shared communicative landscapes' look like?

Is it theoretically possible for congenitally deafblind people to develop language?

Vonen and Nafstad (1999) argue that no tactile language has emerged spontaneously anywhere in the world. Indeed Vonen (2006) presents convincing arguments about why it would be difficult for such a language to emerge. People learning a language needs the perceptual abilities to perceive the language(s) around them and they need to learn from people who already are fluent in those language(s). We can see that for congenitally deafblind people, this will present a significant challenge. They do not have the perceptual abilities to learn spoken or even visually signed languages, due to their hearing and visual impairments. But neither can they find communication partners who are fluent in tactile communication, because none truly exists.[1] So we might conclude that there are insurmountable barriers for congenitally deafblind people developing language.

However, Goldin-Meadow (2005) clearly shows that deaf children of hearing parents, who we might expect to fail to communicate or at most to communicate in non-language-like ways, do develop natural gestures that perform language functions, even in home situations where they cannot perceive the spoken language around them and have not been exposed to sign languages. She argues that they do this by themselves, suggesting some features of language are resilient and that they can develop without outside influence. There is also evidence that a group of deaf Nicaraguan children developed a new fully formed sign language over a 25-year period (Goldin-Meadow 2005; Morford and Kegl 2000; Senghas, Kita and Özyürek 2004), allowing Senghas *et al.* (2004, p.1779) to conclude that 'children naturally possess learning abilities capable of giving language its fundamental structure'. So we could posit that congenitally deafblind people possess these same structures and, like all other children, might be able to develop language without a language model already in existence.

However, language does not just appear from nowhere. Non-linguistic input plays a key role in the acquisition of language. Morford and Kegl (2000) highlight in particular 'homesigns' which may have developed within one family and will only be used by that family. They describe the ways in which groups of deaf children came together, with homesign systems that were different, but out of which language still developed. The circumstances that they identified as being necessary to facilitate this development were:

---

1   It is true that some deaf sign language users who later lose their vision do use very complex and sophisticated tactile sign systems, but these are primarily based on adaptations of their first sign language, as opposed to being fully tactile throughout development.

- ample opportunities for shared communication

- partners willing to communicate in a visuo-spatial modality

- new communication demands associated with preferred
  accommodation to visually oriented deaf partners.

There is immediate relevance here for congenitally deafblind people and
their partners. Congenitally deafblind people will frequently develop id-
iosyncratic gestures, often emerging from movements and actions taken
from activities in which they have participated, so we could imagine that
if there were ample opportunities for shared communication with partners who were willing to communicate in the tactile modality (as opposed
to the auditory or visuo-spatial modalities), then this could lead to new
communication demands. Like the situation with the Nicaraguan
children, we might expect this to flower into language.

Stokoe (2000) hints that perhaps the earliest languages available to
humans were gestural and signed languages. He outlines how a gesture
made by a hand movement may depict things and, at the same time, duplicate features of actions done by or to such things. Thus a gesture 'may
express both noun-like and verb-like meanings and at the same time
show them related' (p.388). He provides wonderful illustrations of how
this might have happened tens of thousands of years ago. For example,
noun phrases 'represented by the symbolism, iconicity or pointing of the
handshape' (p.396) would be subject to adjectival modification depending on what the hand(s) did (e.g. the hands could represent picking up a
'small' jar with hands close together and a 'big' jar with hands further
apart). Similarly, adverbial modifications could be expressed by the face,
the body or the movement of the hands (e.g. if you mime picking up a
hammer and knocking in a nail, depending on the speed of your arm
movement you can express that you did this fast or slowly). Although
Stokoe believes 'all that was needed for the elaboration of the basic
hand-movement structure into full blown syntax existed in the nature of
vision' (p.394), his additional comment that language 'comes from the
body' (p.394) suggests that it could happen tactually, without vision. For
example, with both of a communication partner's hands under a congenitally deafblind person's hands, you could represent lifting a 'big' pot or a
'small' pot, depending on how wide the spread between both hands.
With a congenitally deafblind person's hands on top of a partner's hands,
she could tell you that she hammered in a nail very slowly or very fast,

and this could be done entirely through her gestures and movements, perceived in the tactile medium. It will not necessarily be as quick as telling the story in the visuo-spatial modality and you cannot easily tell the story at a distance, but nevertheless the story can be told.

Where does all this leave us in our thinking about congenitally deafblind people? In many respects we are witnessing the birth of not just a new language but a new mode of language – a language that begins from the perceptual possibilities of the deafblind person (that is to say it is a tactile language) but is then jointly negotiated with communication partners, partners who are willing to move closer to the perceptual world of the deafblind person. This has been affectionately and speculatively termed 'deafblindish' by some (Nafstad and Ask Larssen 2004), and it is a journey that perhaps resembles the flowering of gestural/signed languages millennia ago, when there were no frameworks for pre-existing language models. Concepts such as scaffolding (Wood 1988), guided participation (Rogoff *et al.* 1998), guided construction of knowledge (Mercer 1995) and assisted performance (Tharp and Gallimore 1998) all presuppose that the more competent communication partner is leading the other to his or her preferred language destination. They share a sense of taking someone to a place already known about, teaching skills that others are already expert in, so the responsibility is to take someone's 'hand' and guide that person to a better world. But the practice model that will be described later in this chapter is not one of guidance. It is true that communication partners will know about language, but they will not know about tactile language. So instead, we need to think about a *joint* journey where the negotiation of language is a co-creative process (Nafstad and Rødbroe 1997, 1999) and where the communication partner becomes a 'co-learner' (Brown 2001), attempting to perceive the world from the same touchpoint as the congenitally deafblind person. Communication partners should have a readiness to be the student as well as the teacher (Lane 2003).

Goldin-Meadow (2005) is right that there are some resilient features of language that develop naturally, but she would agree with Vonen (2006) that having other people around is both helpful and necessary for language to develop fully. Congenitally deafblind people can develop language and its starting place lies clearly within their own perceptual experience, but it requires a communication partner who is willing to develop fluency in perceiving the world from a tactile perspective. Interestingly, Rogoff *et al.* (1998) note how infants manage effective communication through tactile contact, because they can perceive slight postural changes when they are carried, so perhaps congenitally deafblind people have never lost these abilities and are already skilled in recognising and using subtle tactile communication strategies. Indeed, for communication partners, perhaps we just need to re-engage with the skills that we all already possess. After all, at key moments in life when words fail us, we know that a hug will still convey a thousand thoughts and emotions.

What are the key features underpinning attitudes and approaches of communication partners?

Despite this theoretical possibility of language emerging for deafblind people, it is the case that linguistic competence has previously been very rarely achieved (Souriau 1990). It is true that part of the reason for this may lie with the nature of congenital deafblindness, where the process of communication could go wrong literally from the moment of birth (Nafstad and Rødbroe 1997; Pease 2000). But it is equally important to recognise the impact that a communication partner's attitude and approach can have on the communicative process (Hart 2003; Rødbroe and Souriau 2000), a point that Trevarthen makes in Chapter 2. Of crucial importance is to recognise the communication and linguistic potential of all congenitally deafblind people. It is too easy just to think of a congenitally deafblind person simply as a person with deficits – without hearing and vision. Instead, we could think of that person more positively, as having touch as his or her pre-eminent source of contact with the external world (Hart 2003). This then helps us to see how communication can be effectively channelled, especially when we think about research that has been done in the field of deafness or blindness. It is the *mismatch* between the communicative modalities of two partners that has a more profound effect on development than does the sensory impairment itself (Bakeman and Adamson 1984; Mohay 1986; Rattray 2000). Thus, the importance of giving the deafblind person a clear, unambiguous message that his or her action, whether that is a movement, gesture or vocalisation, has led to a contingent response on the part of the partner cannot be overstated. (This is a point that Phoebe Caldwell also makes, in Chapter 11, when discussing the intervention of Intensive Interaction.) These messages must be given in a way that is perceivable by the deafblind person. This might be in the tactile medium (including movement, airflow or vibration), but could equally well be through smell or taste (Rødbroe and Souriau 2000).

By responding in a manner that is meaningful to the deafblind person, rather than only to his or her partner, trust can be established between the communication partners. The experience of trusting, or even expecting, that you will receive a response from the other – that you can influence someone else's behaviour – has a fundamental impact on the development of communicative ability (Nafstad and Rødbroe 1999). Just as it is for the human infant, for the deafblind person to receive a matched, or imitative, response from another person helps the deafblind person experience him- or herself as an 'I', even after years of being neglected within social interactions. But it also means the other person is not 'an alien but a kindred spirit – not an "It" but an embryonic "Thou"' (Meltzoff 2002, p.36). This must be equally true for the partner as well. Matching responses to one's partner – imitating – helps to reveal the deafblind person as a 'Thou', thus endowing the deafblind person with a humanity that is often overlooked. Imitation therefore serves the same purpose for the communication partner as it serves for a newborn infant: it shows the other to be just like me (Meltzoff and Moore 1998; Nadel 2002). This is perhaps the real power of imitation for all of the intervention efforts being discussed in this volume: imitation weaves its spell as powerfully on the communication partner as it does on the deafblind person (Heimann 2002; Nadel 2002; Trevarthen 1980).

Putting such insights into practice generated a range of new approaches to deafblind education. Nind and Hewett (1994) developed an imitative technique they labelled Intensive Interaction; Lee and MacWilliams (1995) stressed the importance of co-activity and resonance between two persons' movements; Nafstad and Rødbroe (1999) emphasised the co-creative role that both partners play in negotiating meaning. Two seminal conferences held in Paris in 1996 and 1999 (Deafblind International 1996, 1999) brought practitioners and researchers together to explore emerging perspectives and findings, and these have been followed in recent years by many other publications and research (e.g. Gibson 2005; Janssen 2003; Rødbroe and Souriau 2000; Vege, Bjartvik and Nafstad 2007), all stressing the value of replicating models of child and infant development, where the more competent communicative partner responds contingently, often imitatively, to the actions, gestures and vocalisations of less competent partners. Such exchanges are increasingly regarded as an essential starting point for any communicative partnership. There is a corresponding recognition that if babies are socially precocious from birth (Rosenthal-Rollins 1999) and innate companions and cooperators (Trevarthen 1998), then this must equally be true of deafblind people (Hart 2006; Janssen 2003; Nafstad and Rødbroe 1999; Rødbroe and Souriau 2000). Thus all congenitally deafblind people are potential communication partners. It is of paramount importance that communication partners first grant people this potentiality in order that trusting communicative relationships can develop.

It is important next that communication partners build on the narrative structures that are inherent in early communication episodes, what might be called 'formats' (Bruner 1995), or 'scripts' (Nelson 1985), through which learners come not only to understand more about the cultural context in which they live, but gradually take on increasing responsibility for roles within that script. Whereas at first the learner is akin to an extra in a soap opera, in time she develops as the leading lady in her own blockbuster! Without this opportunity to try new acts, development would cease.

Zeedyk (2006) demonstrates that this has built from early communicative relationships, where it is essential that partners do not know exactly what is coming next. It is this anticipation, the novelty and surprise that keeps both partners interested in the interaction. Caldwell (2006) highlights the importance of surprise when working with people with disabilities, stressing that it should come within the context of a person's existing repertoire. This importance of routines and predictability has long been understood within the deafblind field (Lee and MacWilliams 1995; McInnes and Treffry 1982; Pease 2000), but so too has the need for surprise and novelty, termed by Van Dijk (1989) as 'mismatches', but equivalent to Caldwell's (2006) idea of a 'joke'. Van Dijk calls for routines to be established, with clear starts, middles and ends; when those routines are understood, slight changes should continually be made (i.e. mismatches in expectation), thus giving the learner an opportunity to solve problems as well as an opportunity for expressive communication. Within the context of narrative, it is also important to consider the presence of emotion and dramatic tension, particularly the sense of building any interaction towards a climax and subsequent release of this tension. This makes communication exchanges more memorable and can lead to the formation of what some call Bodily Emotional Traces (Daelman *et al.* 2002).

Examples of such 'traces' have now been captured very clearly in video footage (Daelman *et al.* 1996, 1999a; Vege *et al.* 2007), with movements, gestures and actions clearly coming directly from activities, and those 'traces' themselves becoming the representations of that activity. For example, a famous clip features Thomas, a young deafblind boy, and his teacher playing with a long plastic tunnel (Daelman *et al.* 1999a). The entire interaction is fun for Thomas and leads to a real emotional climax with excited laughter when the teacher goes inside the tunnel and calls to Thomas. Later in the sequence, when Thomas wishes the teacher to go back inside the tunnel, he indicates this by pressing on his cheek and his ear and moving his arm in an action that resembles how his arm had previously been placed over the tunnel. To Thomas, these are the actions and gestures that stick in his mind as most representative and enigmatic of the tunnel episode.

Thomas's actions could be interpreted as declarative communication, where an individual seeks to make a comment or relate an experience to another person. Rødbroe and Souriau (2000) have reported that this was previously rarely seen in deafblind people. There rarely emerged any examples of individuals being able to share feelings or events that were removed from the here-and-now, including wishes for what they would like to do in the future or memories of experiences they had had in the past. Rødbroe and Souriau (2000) have charged that this is because the teaching methods used in the past relied too much on symbolic communicative systems, viewing communication primarily as a means of delivering messages, rather than as a means of people engaging emotionally and psychologically with one another. Rosenthal-Rollins (1999) reports that an over-reliance on instrumental regulation (i.e. imperative communicative function) can have devastating consequences for language acquisition. So one practical implication of this work is that communication partners need to prioritise declarative functions of language over imperative ones (Nafstad and Rødbroe 2007).

The example of Thomas and his teacher also reveals how it is possible to jointly attend to the same external object in a tactile manner. It calls for great sensitivity and observation skills from the communication partner to achieve this joint attention – this meeting of minds – and it depends, says Bruner (1995, p.6), 'not only on a shared or joint focus, but on shared context and shared presuppositions'. This shared context calls for a common touchpoint on the world, and I would suggest also that in developing joint attention it is dependent on the communication partner sharing the interests of the deafblind person. We saw earlier how easy it might be to slip into the trap of imagining that the world for congenitally deafblind people must be a dark and lonely place. Not for them will it be possible to enjoy a crimson-red sunset, or to look out from a mountain top and see a whole landscape of colour and vibrancy unfolding below; never to hear a Mozart symphony or to be awoken on a glorious summer's day with the sound of a bird's chorus.

This is simply wrong. Deafblind people, too, have entire landscapes to behold. The American thinker and teacher, Barbara Miles, offers a much richer, thoughtful vision of deafblind people's worlds. I once saw her pick up a glass, hold it for a moment, and then declare 'Within this glass there is an entire landscape for a deafblind child.' Experienced from the perspective of a tactile 'outfeel' – as opposed to 'outlook' – on the world, it is not difficult to realise the possibilities for wonder and awe in such everyday objects. Lane (2003) sets us a challenge 'to find ways to re-organize our daily interactions that are attuned to vision and hearing so that they become attuned instead to touch'.

It is important that communication partners discover this tactile landscape that is the focus of the deafblind person's interest, bearing in mind Prechtel's words that 'the highest form of praise is to acknowledge a person's interests and to explore the world together' (Miles 2006). Miles (2006) demonstrated one example of this through video footage of a young deafblind boy and his teacher in an Indian classroom. On the first day we see the young boy coming into the school, with the teacher encouraging him to take part in his normal morning routine of going round other classrooms and offices to find out who was there and to say hello. This was all in the interests of developing his social and communication skills. We see that the young boy's interest is taken by various objects along this journey, and he employs his residual vision to gaze at clocks, computers and papers lying on desks. Each time he does this, the teacher draws his attention back to the task of saying 'good morning' to the people he meets on his journey. On the second day of filming the teacher has been advised simply to follow the interests of the boy and to engage in joint exploration of whatever he shows an interest in. As he walks into the school and the teacher greets him, the boy looks towards the ring on his teacher's finger. The teacher touches the ring and encourages the boy to do so as well. Within a short time they are both seated on the floor in the school corridor and they are jointly exploring the ring together, their hands constantly overlapping with each other as they feel and touch the ring. Both seem lost in each other's company and both are fully engaged in the exploration of the ring. They are lost in the kind of intensive inter-action that Coia and Jardine Handley describe so eloquently in Chapter 7. Sharing the interests and landscapes of communicatively impaired partners is of such paramount importance because joint attention is seen by some as the gateway to language (Butterworth 1995), through its creation of what Bruner (1995) terms 'shared social realities', what I prefer to think of as 'shared communicative landscapes'.

What would an intervention designed to develop these 'shared communicative landscapes' look like?

The previous section might now suggest an 'ideal' communication exchange between a congenitally deafblind person and his or her com-munication partners, where we see:

- real trust and relationship existing – the fundamentals of communication are in place

- there is close, physical proximity between the two partners – we could describe it as intimate

- overall the activity has a narrative structure, with a clear start, middle and end and a sense of building to a climax before releasing the tension

- routines developing and a sense of anticipation built by mismatch, novelty and surprise, which will have been present from the earliest communication exchanges

- real drama emerge from the exchange, through exaggerating emotions, movements and gestures

- joint exploration of objects with maximum attention being drawn to the tactile features of the environment

- both partners aware of each other's involvement in the activity and jointly attending to the same features

- both partners make reference to the activity and what is happening. They will do this as they undertake the activity, but also afterwards that same day and even in subsequent days.

Let us now imagine a congenitally deafblind person and his or her communication partner going for a walk in the park. Imagine that there is clear agreement that the occasion – the walk – has begun, an agreement that could be achieved by always starting at the same tree. Imagine that both partners fully explore this tree. They do not just stand back and admire it from a distance, but instead, both sets of hands weave with each other in a dance of exploration and stimulation, feeling the texture of the bark, running fingers along the soft, velvety ridges, discovering the spongy moss that it is growing on the side, pressing it, feeling it with their fingers, their palms, their knuckles, letting it bounce gently back against their hands as they establish a rhythmic pulse on the side of the tree. Imagine that after this prologue a whole series of events is anticipated by both partners, because they are following a route that is familiar to them, having been jointly negotiated on earlier occasions.

This occasion does not have to be imagined, for this description represents precisely the work in which we are engaged in Sense Scotland, an organisation that supports deafblind people. One of my colleagues in Sense Scotland, Dr Joe Gibson, has developed the kind of route I have just described, in collaboration with one of the deafblind men we support, whom I will call here Joshua. It takes in five trees which act as clear markers for where they are on the route. First they explore a holly tree, then a tree with a strange branch formation that they have come to 'refer' to as the 'over-under tree' because to get around the tree you have first to climb over one branch and then duck under another. Then there is the 'old tree with the moss', then the 'tree with the skin', where the bark has come off over the years. Finally there is the 'tree that has fallen over in the wind'. Here they are able to explore its roots (re-christened as its feet, an easier concept for deafblind people to grasp). There are other set events that take place on the walk: a conversation at the start of the walk that outlines the route they will take, coffee that is drunk half way along the journey, a conversation that takes place at the end. Other events also of course happen, including unplanned ones, which adds to the drama and narrative of the occasion, and which facilitate Joshua's understanding of the world around him. One week, it will be a boot lace that comes undone; another week it will be the cake they eat instead of a biscuit; sometimes it will be raining and other times sunny, and this will make the path muddy or dry. All of these elements can have attention directed to them. Sometimes, Joshua will discover something that takes his interest – a leaf that has fallen onto the branch he is exploring or some moss that has come away from the tree in his hand. It is Joe's role as his communication partner to share these interests and to endorse Joshua's attention in them, by engaging in that attention himself.

Whatever Joshua's interest is drawn to, the actions and movements associated with exploring that object can be exaggerated. For example, in discovering a leaf by chance, both partners can work together to reach higher and higher up the tree to feel for other leaves, thus leaving an imprint of the activity in the minds of both partners. And talking about these activities should not just be left to certain times but should intrude into all parts of the walk. As an interesting new leaf is discovered, the word 'leaf' can be fingerspelled right there, it can be explored, Joe can share Joshua's emotion. Does this make us feel excited and happy, or is the leaf horrible to touch because it is is cold and wet? Is it like the one we touched earlier, or is it different? This is an interaction permeated by communication, engagement, emotion, and ultimately by language.

Engaging in this process, however, means slowing the world down. It means a full and complete immersion in the experience. It means letting the trees come to you as much as you come to them! Thich Nhat Hanh (1995, p.21) recounts, in his book on the practice of mindfulness, asking a group of children to peel a tangerine slowly, 'noticing the mist and the fragrance of the tangerine and then bringing it up to [your] mouth and having a mindful bite, in full awareness of the texture and taste of the fruit and the juice coming out... When you peel it and smell it, it's wonderful. You can take your time eating a tangerine and be very happy.' Communication partners can take this same approach when exploring the world alongside a deafblind person. Parents who use imitative responsiveness with their child with autism are also essentially slowing down and immersing themselves in the moment, as described by O'Neill, Jones and Zeedyk in Chapter 4, just as are those care staff who use 'Adaptive Interaction' in their work with elderly people with dementia, as described by Ellis and Astell in Chapter 8. Think, here, of the trees not simply from a seeing–hearing perspective, but from a tactile and bodily perspective. This is how a 'shared communicative landscape' is created, along with the Bodily Emotional Traces that such exploration leaves – those movements, actions and gestures that are remembered alongside the emotional content of an activity. These traces lay the foundations for negotiated, shared meaning between congenitally deafblind people and their partners (Daelman *et al.* 2002; Gibson 2005) – and perhaps for all of us, from the time when we were infants and were first negotiating the world around us with our caregivers.

Conclusion

This chapter has set out to establish that there is no theoretical, or indeed practical, reason why congenitally deafblind people should not develop language. It has highlighted a range of key ideas that help underpin the attitudes and approaches that need to be adopted by the communication partner. Crucially, they should be prepared to develop trusting relationships with the deafblind person, and they should strive to 'feel' the world from a tactile perspective, aligning their attention to the interests of the deafblind person. When this basis is used to negotiate joint activities that have clear structure, and a declarative function, then the foundations for shared language are in place. Across the world we are now seeing such ideas emerge in our practical work with deafblind people (Ask Larssen 2007; Vege *et al.* 2007). We are venturing into a world where congenitally deafblind people can move away from the here-and-now to tell their own stories, not just to one communication partner, but to new partners that they meet in new places. It is an exciting time to be working in this field.

It perhaps seems a paradox that in order to talk about events in the past, it is first necessary to share communicative landscapes fully in the present. This is reminiscent of Buber's own realisation – of the importance of experiencing each moment 'as a moment in and of itself, without judging it based on the past with its wounds or the future with its uncertainties' (cited in Mayhall and Mayhall 2004, p.18). Communication partners must fully immerse themselves in the present with their deafblind partner, making the absolute most of this moment and the next moment and the next. This apparent contradiction will make it much easier for that moment to be recalled, and generalised from, at some future moment. There is a sense that we are (re-)presenting the past at some point in the future. By that I mean we make the past come alive (or present) again. In order to make this possible, the deafblind field – and all the rest of us as well – should not be too concerned about future conversations while we are undertaking activities of the present.

Barbara Miles' beautiful words from her poem 'Solstice Meadow' perhaps sum this up more succinctly:

May we carry whatever seeds are ours to carry
into some remembered morning
yet to come.

References

Ask Larssen, F. (2007) 'The Washing-Smooth Hole-Fish and other findings of semantic potential and negotiation strategies in conversation with congenitally deafblind children.' MA thesis in Cognitive Semiotics, Center for Semiotics, University of Aarhus 2003. *Communication Network Update Series No. 9.* Nordic Staff Training Centre for Deafblind Services (www.nud.dk).

Bakeman, R. and Adamson, L.B. (1984) 'Co-ordinating attention to people and objects in mother/infant and peer/infant interactions.' *British Journal of Developmental Psychology 4,* 43–49.

Brown, N. (2001) 'Communication with congenitally deafblind people.' Presentation at Deafblind International seminar. Suresnes, Paris, 2–6 May.

Bruner, J. (1995) 'From Joint Attention to the Meeting of Minds: An Introduction.' In C. Moore and P.J. Dunham (eds) *Joint Attention: Its Origins and Role in Development.* Hillsdale, NJ: Lawrence Erlbaum Associates.

Butterworth, G. (1995) 'Origins of mind in perception and action.' In C. Moore and P.J. Dunham (eds) *Joint Attention: Its Origins and Role in Development.* Hillsdale, NJ: Lawrence Erlbaum Associates.

Caldwell, P. (2006) 'Speaking the other's language: Imitation as a gateway to relationship.' *Infant and Child Development 15,* 3, 275–282.

Daelman, M., Janssen, M., Ask Larssen, F., Nafstad, A., Rødbroe, I., Souriau, J. and Visser, A. (2002) 'Update on the concept of blending in relation to congenital deafblindness and the formation of meaning in communicative interactions.' *Communication Network Update Series No.4.* Nordic Staff Training Centre for Deafblind Services (www.nud.dk).

Daelman, M., Nafstad, A., Rødbroe, I., Visser, T. and Souriau, J. (1996) *The emergence of communication. Contact and interaction patterns. Persons with congenital deafblindness.* IAEDB working group on communication. Suresnes, France: CNEFEI. Video.

Daelman, M., Nafstad, A., Rødbroe, I., Visser, T. and Souriau, J. (eds) (1999a) *The Emergence of Communication – Part II.* IAEDB working group on communication. Suresnes, France: CNEFEI. Video.

Daelman, M., Nafstad, A., Rødbroe, I., Souriau, J. and Visser, A. (eds) (1999b) *The Emergence of Communication – Part II.* Paris: Centre National du Suresnes.

Deafblind International (1996) 'Communication and congenital deafblindness. The development of communication. What's new?' Conference Suresnes, Paris, France, 23–26 June.

Deafblind International (1999) 'The development of communication in persons with congenital deafblindness.' Conference Suresnes, Paris, France, 11–14 April.

Gibson, J. (2005) 'Climbing to communicate: An investigation into the experiences of congenitally deafblind adults who have participated in outdoor education.' Thesis presented in part fulfilment of the requirements for the degree of Doctor of Philosophy, University of Strathclyde, Glasgow.

Goldin-Meadow, S. (2005) *The Resilience of Language – What Gesture Creation in Deaf Children Can Tell Us about How All Children Learn Language.* New York: Psychology Press.

Hart, P. (2003) 'The role of a partner in communication episodes with a deafblind person.' *Deafblind Review 31*, 4–7.

Hart, P. (2006) 'Using imitation with congenitally deafblind adults: Establishing meaningful communication partnerships.' *Infant and Child Development 15*, 3, 263–274.

Heimann, M. (2002) 'Notes on Individual Differences and the Assumed Elusiveness of Neo-natal Imitation.' In A.N. Meltzoff and W. Prinz (eds) *The Imitative Mind: Development, Evolution, and Brain Bases.* Cambridge: Cambridge University Press.

Janssen, M.J. (2003) 'Fostering harmonious interactions between deafblind children and their educators.' PhD thesis, University of Nimejan, Netherlands.

Kugiumutzakis, G. (1998) 'Neonatal imitation in the intersubjective companion space.' In S. Bråten (ed.) *Intersubjective Communication and Emotion in Early Ontogeny.* Cambridge: Cambridge University Press.

Lane, H. (2003) 'Afterword.' In B. Miles, *Talking the Language of the Hands to the Hands.* Accessed 21/02/08 at www.dblink.org/lib/hands.htm.

Lee, M. and MacWilliams, L. (1995) *Movement, Gesture and Sign: An Interactive Approach to Sign Communication for Children who are Visually Impaired with Additional Disabilities.* Edinburgh: RNIB.

Mayhall, C.W. and Mayhall, T.B. (2004) *On Buber.* Toronto: Wadsworth.

McInnes, J.M. and Treffry, J.A. (1982) *Deafblind Infants and Children: A Developmental Guide.* Toronto: University of Toronto Press.

Meltzoff, A.N. (2002) 'Elements of a Developmental Theory of Imitation.' In A.N. Meltzoff and W. Prinz (eds) *The Imitative Mind: Development, Evolution, and Brain Bases.* Cambridge: Cambridge University Press.

Meltzoff, A.N. and Moore, M.K. (1998) 'Infant Intersubjectivity: Broadening the Dialogue to Include Imitation, Identity and Intention.' In S. Bråten (ed.) *Intersubjective Communication and Emotion in Early Ontogeny.* Cambridge: Cambridge University Press.

Mercer, N. (1995) *The Guided Construction of Knowledge: Talk Amongst Teachers and Learners.* Clevedon: Multilingual Matters Ltd.

Miles, B. (2006) 'Exploring the world together: Talking the language of the hands.' Presentation at Sense Scotland Seminar: Partners in Communication – An International Perspective, 13 January 2006, Glasgow.

Mohay, H. (1986) 'The adjustment of maternal conversation to hearing and hearing impaired children: A twin study.' *Journal of the British Association of Teachers of the Deaf 10*, 2, 37–44.

Morford, J.P. and Kegl, J.A. (2000) 'Gestural Precursors to Linguistic Constructs: How Input Shapes the Form of Language.' In D. McNeill (ed.) *Language and Gesture.* Cambridge: Cambridge University Press.

Nadel, J. (2002) 'Imitation and Imitation Recognition: Functional Use in Preverbal Infants and Nonverbal Children with Autism.' In A.N. Meltzoff and W. Prinz (eds) *The Imitative Mind: Development, Evolution, and Brain Bases.* Cambridge: Cambridge University Press.

Nafstad, A.V. and Ask Larssen, F. (2004) 'The relation between potential and realized meaning.' *Communication Network Update Series No. 5.* Nordic Staff Training Centre for Deafblind Services (www.nud.dk).

Nafstad, A. and Rødbroe, I. (1997) 'Congenital Deafblindness, Interaction and Development towards a Model of Intervention.' In M. Laurent (ed.) *Communication and Congenital Deafblindness. The Development of Communication. What is New?* Suresnes, France: Editions du Centre National de Suresnes.

Nafstad, A. and Rødbroe, I. (1999) *Co-creating Communication.* Oslo: Forlaget-Nord Press.

Nafstad, A. and Rødbroe, I. (2007) 'Co-creating communication with persons with congenital deafblindness.' *Communication Network Update Series No. 8.* Nordic Staff Training Centre for Deafblind Services (www.nud.dk).

Nelson, K. (1985) *Making Sense: The Acquisition of Shared Meaning.* New York: Academic.

Nhat Hanh, T. (1995) *Peace is Every Step: The Path of Mindfulness in Everyday Life.* London: Rider.

Nind, M. and Hewett, D. (1994) *Access to Communication: Developing the Basics of Communication with People with Severe Learning Difficulties through Intensive Interaction.* London: David Fulton Publishers.

Pease, L. (2000) 'Creating a Communicating Environment.' In S. Aitken, M. Buultjens, C. Clark, J.T. Eyre and L. Pease (eds) *Teaching Children who are Deafblind.* London: David Fulton Publishers.

Rattray, J. (2000) 'Dancing in the dark: The effects of visual impairment on the nature of early mother/infant dyadic interactions and communication.' PhD thesis, University of Dundee.

Reddy, V. (2003) 'On being the object of attention: implications for self–other consciousness.' *Trends in Cognitive Sciences 7,* 397–402.

Rødbroe, I. and Souriau, J. (2000) 'Communication.' In J.M. McInnes (ed.) *A Guide to Planning and Support for Individuals who are Deafblind.* Toronto: University of Toronto Press.

Rogoff, B., Mosier, C., Mistry, J. and Göncü, A. (1998) 'Toddlers guided participation with their caregivers in cultural activity.' In M. Woodhead, D. Faulkner and K. Littleton (eds) *Cultural Worlds of Early Childhood.* London: Routledge.

Rosenthal-Rollins, P. (1999) 'Pragmatics in Early Interaction and Beginning of Language.' In M. Daelman, A. Nafstad, I. Rødbroe, J. Souriau and A. Visser (eds) *The Emergence of Communication – Part II.* Paris: Centre National du Suresnes.

Sacks, O. (1995) 'To See and not See.' In *An Anthropologist on Mars.* New York: Vintage.

Senghas, A., Kita, S. and Özyürek, A. (2004) 'Children creating core properties of language; evidence from an emerging sign language in Nicaragua.' *Science 305,* 1779–1782.

Souriau, J. (1990) 'The development of language.' *Deafblind Education 6,* 5–8.

Stokoe, W. (2000) 'Gesture to Sign (Language).' In D. McNeill (ed.) *Language and Gesture.* Cambridge: Cambridge University Press.

Tharp, R. and Gallimore, R. (1998) 'A Theory of Learning as Assisted Performance.' In D. Faulkner, K. Littleton and M. Woodhead (eds) *Learning Relationships in the Classroom.* London: Routledge.

Trevarthen, C. (1980) 'The foundations of intersubjectivity: Development of interpersonal and cooperative understanding in infants.' In D.R. Olson (ed.) *The Social Foundation of Language and Thought: Essays in Honor of Jerome Bruner.* New York: Norton.

Trevarthen, C. (1998) 'The Concept and Foundations of Infant Intersubjectivity.' In S. Bråten (ed.) *Intersubjective Communication and Emotion in Early Ontogeny.* Cambridge: Cambridge University Press.

Van Dijk, J. (1989) *The Sint-Michelgestel Approach to Diagnosis and Education of Multisensory Impaired Persons.* St Michelsgestel, Netherlands: Institut Voor Doven.

Vege, G., Bjartvik, R.F. and Nafstad, A. (2007) *Traces.* DVD. Andebu Dovblindcenter, Norway.

Vonen, A.M. (2006) 'Access to the language of the culture.' Presentation at NUD conference: Co-Creating Communication with Persons with Congenital Deafblindness, 29 April 2006, Oslo, Norway.

Vonen, A.M. and Nafstad, A. (1999) 'The Concept of Natural Language: What Does this Mean for Deafblind People?' In M. Daelman, A. Nafstad, I. Rødbroe, J. Souriau and A. Visser (eds) *The Emergence of Communication – Part II.* Paris: Centre National du Suresnes.

Wood, D. (1988) *How Children Think and Learn.* Oxford: Blackwell.

Zeedyk, M.S. (2006) 'From intersubjectivity to subjectivity: The transformative roles of emotional intimacy and imitation.' *Infant and Child Development 15,* 321–344.

CHAPTER 6

USING IMITATION TO ESTABLISH CHANNELS OF COMMUNICATION WITH INSTITUTIONALISED CHILDREN IN ROMANIA: BRIDGING THE GAP

Clifford E. Davies, M. Suzanne Zeedyk, Sarah Walls, Naomi Betts and Sarah Parry

In 2006 the lead authors of this chapter made two visits to a privately run day-care centre in the Romanian town of Slatina, where we used imitative interaction (often refered to as Intensive Interaction) as a means of making communicative contact with children with language impairments. Our preliminary results have been very promising and, in this chapter, we report on the effects of our intervention on both the children and their caregivers.

Institutional care in Romania

When the communist regime of Ceaucescu fell in 1990 the shameful condition of Romanian institutional child-care provision was revealed. State control of fertility regulation had resulted in a very large number of babies, particularly those born with any form of handicap, being abandoned by families who were simply too poor to look after them, and these children were then reared in overcrowded orphanages where staff did little more than keep their charges alive (Langton 2006).

In the following years many such children were adopted into families in Europe and North America, and their developmental progress monitored by researchers (Chisholm *et al.* 1998; O'Connor *et al.* 2000). These children provided researchers with a rare, if unfortunate, opportunity to study the effects (and reversibility) of deprivation in what has been called the 'ultimate experiment' (Talbot 1998).

In recent years the Romanian government, motivated in part by the need to meet criteria set for entry into the EU, has taken considerable steps to improve the standard of care afforded to abandoned children. Many areas of the country are still experiencing severe difficulties in providing an appropriate level of care (Gloviczki 2004), however. This is particularly true for those children who, when assessed at three years of age, are classified as 'irrecuperable' and placed into a stream of the child-care system that accentuates their disabled status. As a result, many children growing up in the Romanian child-care system still suffer a triple handicap – they have been born with a mental or physical disability, have been abandoned by their parents and then experience a lifetime of chronic neglect in state care thereafter. These children often present with communicative difficulties so extreme that they can be described as 'quasi-autistic' (Rutter *et al.* 1999).

Interventions with Romanian orphans

Early studies of institutional care in Romania (e.g. Kaler and Freeman 1994) demonstrated cognitive delays and serious impairments in social functioning in young children, associated with poor standards of child-care by under-trained staff. More recent studies (e.g. Smyke *et al.* 2007) in large part replicated these findings, but also reported that differences in the caregiving environment were associated with differences in outcomes, particularly in terms of social and cognitive functioning and behavioural conduct. An educational intervention study by Sparling *et al.* (2005), working with institutionalised Romanian children under the age of three, was able to show substantial growth in measures of personal–social development, fine motor-adaptive skills, gross motor development and language by introducing stable adult–child relationships, small group sizes and a protocol of enriched caregiving and educational activities. Their major conclusion was that 'the behaviour of caregivers is crucial since their behaviour carries the intervention to the children'.

In the early 1990s many Romanian children were adopted into the United States, Canada and Great Britain, and have been the subject of much research interest. The English and Romanian Adoptees (ERA) study team, headed by Professor Michael Rutter, was able to show that children adopted under the age of six months were able to make substantial physical and cognitive recoveries and, at age four years, were faring as well as British children adopted within the UK (Rutter *et al.* 1998). Older adoptees also showed substantial improvements, but were more likely to have persistent cognitive, socio-emotional and health problems, although there was great variability in the extent to which individual children were affected by their early institutional experiences (Rutter *et al.* 2001). Very similar findings were reported for children adopted into Canadian homes (Fisher *et al.* 1997; Morrison and Ellwood 2000).

The interventions described above have all focused on institutionalised Romanian children from the 'normal' orphanages. To our knowledge, there are no reports in the academic literature of remedial intervention being carried out with children classified as 'irrecuperable' in Romania.

Imitation and Intensive Interaction

Ever since Meltzoff and Moore (1977) published their classic demonstration of infants' imitation of facial gestures, the ability to imitate has been seen by some as a benchmark of human-ness. Indeed, Csibra and Gergely (2005) have argued that pedagogy (and the consequent transmission of culture) in part depends upon our willingness and ability to imitate the behaviours of others. Imitation, then, permits links to be forged between individuals, which would lead to the conclusion that an impairment in imitative ability might explain the psychological failure to connect with others which is so characteristic of people with autism (Meltzoff and Gopnik 1993).

In most human interactions, however, the roles of imitator and imitatee are interchanged reciprocally, so that each individual takes turns fulfilling each role and, while much theory and research has been devoted to what it means to imitate, much less has focused on what it means to be *imitated* (but see Nadel 2002; Nadel *et al.* 2004; Zeedyk 2006). Spontaneous imitation can be readily observed in mother–infant interactions (Rochat 2007), and the interchangeability of roles may facilitate referential communication. Spontaneous imitation has also been observed between young people with learning difficulties and their caregivers (e.g. O'Neill and Zeedyk 2006), although the role of imitator does not seem to be equally divided between partners and was more often adopted by the carers.

The concept of using the basic mechanism of imitation as a means of communicating purposefully with impaired individuals was first introduced by Ephraim (1986), who named the technique 'Augmented Mothering'. It has since proved to be a successful therapeutic technique for opening a channel of communication with individuals with communication difficulties, and is now more often referred to as 'Intensive Interaction' (Caldwell 2006; Nind and Hewett 1994). Over the past decade, the intervention of Intensive Interaction has gained increasing attention as a means of enhancing the social abilities of individuals with severe communicative impairments. It provides a pre-eminent example of what has come to be known in the fields of special needs education (Garner, Hinchcliffe and Sandow 1995) and multiple sensory impairment (e.g. Van den Tillart 2000) as an 'interactive' or 'reciprocal' approach.

The theoretical and practical base of Intensive Interaction is informed by knowledge about the nature of parent–infant communication (e.g. Beebe *et al.* 1985; Stern 1985; Trevarthen 1978), in which sensitive, reciprocal responses from a caregiver are seen as the foundation from which all interpersonal skills emerge. The central aim of Intensive Interaction is to establish rapport with clients, by using their own movements and behaviours in a reciprocal, responsive manner. The familiarity of those actions renders them meaningful to the client, thus creating the joint context necessary for communicative exchanges. Intensive Interaction contrasts with more traditional behavioural approaches, which focus on behaviours themselves, rather than their meaning for the individual, and which seek to change those behaviours deemed to be 'undesirable' or 'non-adaptive', rather than valuing them as significant to that person. Some empirical evaluations of Intensive Interaction's effects on social and communicative development have been carried out (e.g. Nind 1996; Nind and Kellett 2002; Watson and Fisher 1997; Zeedyk, Caldwell and Davies 2007). Most of this work has focused on reported work with small samples; no large scale, well-controlled studies of Intensive Interaction have yet been carried out (and indeed, many practitioners would argue this is impracticable). Most evaluations of imitative techniques have also worked with trained practitioners. Only a few have reported on efforts to work with non-specialists (usually parents, e.g. Ingersoll and Gergans 2007; O'Neill 2006). The study reported here contrasted with both of these trends; we attempted to work with a larger sample (18 children) and to train volunteers in the use of Intensive Interaction.

The design of this study

The work reported here is part of a larger study on the effectiveness of Intensive Interaction that we have recently initiated in Romania, working with children with severe communicative impairments. We were working with a specialist day-care centre, entitled Casa Luminii (House of Light), run by a charitable organisation, which provides an enhanced, individualised developmental programme for a small proportion of children in the local area. The children, aged approximately 4 to 15 years, are in state care and have all been classified as 'irrecuperable', having been orphaned or abandoned by parents due to fears of developmental or medical abnormalities. These include disorders that are commonly associated with socio-communicative difficulties (e.g. autism, cerebral palsy, blindness), as well as abnormalities that, in other cultures, would be regarded as temporary or even unrelated to socio-communicative problems (e.g. cleft or lip palate, physical handicaps, visual squint). No standard developmental inventories or diagnoses were available for the children, and whatever the nature of their initial disorders, the developmental trajectories for all of them had been severely compromised by the poor care they had received in state institutions. The children in the sample with whom we were working here typically had no language, were severely socially withdrawn, frequently engaged in self-harm (e.g. biting their hand, scratching their face or body, hitting their head), and many also had difficulties at some point in walking or feeding themselves unaided. These are typical symptoms of what is now known as 'institutional autism' (Federici 1999; Rutter et al. 2001; Spitz 1945). Intensive Interaction is very well suited to such behavioural challenges, and we therefore expected the technique would benefit the children, although this was, to our knowledge, the first time that this technique had been utilised in a Romanian setting.

The 18 children with whom we worked (ten girls and eight boys) all attend the Casa Luminii day-care centre for 20 hours per week (four hours each morning over five days), and have been doing so between six months and five years. The aim of the centre is to nurture the children's development such that their chance of being fostered or adopted by local Romanian families is increased. An important element of the Casa Luminii programme involves the visits of young people (aged 16 to 18 years) who work closely with the children, on a voluntary basis, for two-week periods. Such visits take place approximately ten times during the year (with different groups of volunteers). The young people raise funds for the centre, in exchange for which they gain experience of providing one-to-one attention for the children. They are not trained in specialist techniques, but are simply encouraged to play as affectionately and spontaneously with the children as possible. The opportunities offered by this programme are clearly prized by the volunteers. They feel they benefit at a professional level, given that many are considering careers in the special needs or medical fields, but more importantly they benefit at a personal level, as a consequence of working so intensely with the children on a daily basis.

In the present study we took advantage of this setting to train the volunteers in the basic precepts of Intensive Interaction, so that this could be incorporated into their methods of working with the children. None of them had previous familiarity with or training in the approach. We gave them a brief training session in Intensive Interaction, and then simply encouraged them to try it with the children. While this training format is somewhat unusual, in that it does not follow the comprehensive training curriculum that is available for Intensive Interaction (e.g. Nind and Hewett 1994, 2001), it is entirely in keeping with the wider range of approaches that have now been employed to introduce practitioners, parents, carers and special needs staff to Intensive Interaction, including one-to-one training sessions, books and video instruction materials.

The volunteer practitioners were each allocated to the care of a particular child, and asked to work with that child as often as possible for the rest of the week. We recorded a series of short (five-minute) videotapes of each of the practitioners working with their allocated child. These initial sessions were classed as 'standard play'. We then provided the imitation training to all volunteers, and asked them to incorporate this method of interaction into all their subsequent interactions with children. We again recorded five minutes of play for each child and volunteer, and classed this as 'imitative play'. In their interactions the children and volunteers were able to make use of any of the play equipment that was available at the centre, and were free to play either indoors in the playroom or outside in the playground or gardens.

Each of the recorded sessions was later coded in detail for the occurrence of two key social behaviours: eye gaze and touch. Eye gaze was defined as any time when the child's eyes were directed toward the volunteer's face. Touch was defined as any time when the child instigated physical contact with the volunteer. The standard and imitation sessions were coded separately by different coders who were not aware of the purpose of the study at that time. We recorded the amount of time that each child spent engaged in these two behaviours, in the two types of play. We expected that levels of engagement would be higher during the imitation sessions compared with the standard sessions.

Quantitative analyses

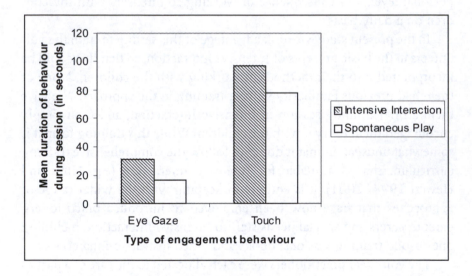

Figure 6.1: Mean duration of eye gaze and touch during five-minute sessions of standard and imitative play (averaged over 16 children)

The mean durations of eye gaze and physical contact for both standard and imitation sessions are shown in Figure 6.1. Only 16 children were included in the quantitative analyses, due to equipment problems.

It can be seen that both eye gaze and physical contact occurred more often in the imitation condition. However, this difference was statistically significant only for eye gaze (t(15) = 2.12, p <.05); it was non-significant for physical contact (t(15) =0.67; n/s.). This indicates that when volunteers responded imitatively to the children's behaviour, it had a reliably positive impact on their gaze to their partner. Although touching also increased for the group as a whole, it did not change sufficiently to allow the difference to be attributed to the volunteers' style of responding.

Another way of looking at these data is to determine the number of children whose engagement changed between the two sessions. How many children showed an increase in engagement during imitative sessions (as compared to standard sessions) and how many children showed a decrease? On the measure of eye gaze, this ratio was 11:3 (with two others who showed no change at all). That distribution is highly unlikely to have occurred by chance (Fisher exact probability = 0.038), so the difference can be attributed to the intervention. On the physical contact measure, however, the ratio was 9:5 (again, with two who showed no change), which is not statistically significant (Fisher exact probability = 0.208). It seems, then, that the use of imitative responsiveness did have an impact on the children's gaze to their partners, but it had no impact on their physical contact with them.

Qualitative analyses

At the end of the study we asked the volunteers to write an account reflecting on their experiences of using the Intensive Interaction approach. The contents of these accounts were then systematically analysed, using the qualitative technique of thematic analysis (see Zeedyk, Davies, Parry and Caldwell 2007 for a more detailed account). What the volunteers said accorded with the quantitative findings, and also provided insights into how the trainees experienced Intensive Interaction.

All 12 of the participating volunteers reported observing positive changes in engagement in the children they worked with, citing a variety of behaviours as evidence of this shift.[1]

One of the most frequently cited behaviours was an increase in the children's *attention to their partner.*

> Before we were told about imitation, all I had seen of Mircea was him hugging somebody, making limited [communicative] contact. With seconds of trying imitation, he was looking up at me and communicating more, by clicking his tongue, blowing rasp-

---

1   In the quotes provided, the names of all children have been changed in order to protect their anonymity. The identity of the volunteer who made the comment is indicated by the numeric identifier provided at the end of the quote.

berries, and smiling. This continued for the hour that he stayed at the Centre with me. I kept up imitation for the duration. [5]

Beatrice has a tendency to stand by herself and do nothing. On a couple of occasions I imitated her mouth, head and hand movements. This caused her to look at me, and to go on to imitate my own hand movements. I had previously been unable to encourage her to engage with me at all. [7]

Another behavioural indicator was an increase in the amount of *positive affect* displayed by the children.

Even more amazingly, the next day, while pushing Ramona on the swing, several of us were imitating her, and she became more animated in her noises, and laughed and giggled for longer than she has previously been known to do. [6]

When we first arrived at the Centre, Serghei would not interact with any other children or helpers in any way. He would spend his time sitting alone and bouncing a plastic ball or similar object. No amount of encouragement would bring Serghei out of his 'own fantasy world'... I was surprised to see that Serghei responded extremely well [to imitation] and seemed to come out of his shell. He started to run around the garden, laughing and smiling and interacting well. He was paying attention to movements and vocalisations, and responding. [8]

A third primary means through which increased social engagement was perceived in the children was via an increase in their *proximity to others*.

Brindusa is a very boisterous girl who loves to run around, be picked up, be on your shoulders, or be on the swings. She doesn't usually like to be on your lap or to play games other than running around. However, when I introduced imitation this all changed. I began our play as usual by running up and down the garden with her, but this time I imitated every sound and facial expression she made, and I made sure that she heard and saw what I was doing. After about 30 seconds, she stopped, pushed me down so that I was sitting on the grass, and sat on my lap. We began to have a conversation with the sound 'aah'. I would wait for her to say it, and then I would respond. I developed this into a sort of anticipation game where sometimes I would on purpose not say anything, in order to tease her. This resulted in her getting really excited and trying to force my mouth open into an 'aah' shape. She absolutely loved this game and every time I would give in and eventually say 'aah', she would give me the tightest hug and laugh. [3]

Ion now places his head on my lap, and spends a lot less time in his trances. [9]

Finally, *increased flexibility and ease in interactions* seemed to provide a particularly strong indicator of increased engagement.

I found that imitation worked very well with Madalina, and she interacts much more with me during and after the imitation session. This meant it was easier to get her to do things. [2]

The clapping can be used as a means to an end. You can do whatever you want with Andrei, as long as you have the clapping rhythm. [11]

This last signal may have been particularly significant for the volunteers because increased flexibility permitted the *spontaneous creation of new games and routines*. These games always included elements introduced by the children. Significantly, the two elements most commonly cited as having been introduced into these spontaneous games are predicted by Intensive Interaction theory. The first of these elements was *testing or teasing* on the part of the child, as if he or she wished to make sure that this new partner could be trusted to 'really get it right'.

Monica noticed my imitation of her hands almost immediately, and would change them as if testing my ability to copy her. [6]

Roxana is a very frightened and untrusting girl, who is difficult to engage with and who often lashes out violently at the other children and staff at the centre. She often rocks back and forth in frustration, so I decided to stand next to Roxana and imitate her rocking. When she noticed me doing this, she started smiling, and continued to watch me while she was rocking. The rocking then turned into a sort of game, with Roxana purposely rocking in different ways, her watching me imitate her, and her smiling with enjoyment. I enjoyed playing this game very much, as I had never been able to play a game with Roxana before, and I got greater

satisfaction out of working with Roxana when she was engaging
with me and enjoying herself. [7]

The second element of the new games involved the *child imitating the
adult's actions*, as if to demonstrate that he or she fully understood how this
new game was played.

> There have been several times during the week where Nela has
> chosen to imitate me. For example, if she sees me starting to fill up
> the teapot with sand, she will join in too. One time she also imi-
> tated one of the other boys, when he was jumping down the stairs
> in a particular way. [1]

> The imitation with Paula turned into a game, with her purposely
> making large movements for me to imitate, and her laughing
> when I did. She would now even copy movements that I made,
> and we imitated each other back and forth for about an hour. [7]

Overall, it is clear that the kinds of behavioural shifts predicted in the
Intensive Interaction literature were observed by the volunteers. They
had been given no particular instructions about what should be included
in their accounts, and yet they gave repeated examples of the same kinds
of changes that have been cited elsewhere. Moreover, wherever the volunteers mentioned the amount of time that had been required for such
shifts to emerge, the period cited was a matter of minutes or even seconds.
This accords with the authors' own informal impressions of the interactions between the volunteers and children, and is supported by other,
more detailed work (e.g. Caldwell 2005; Zeedyk, Caldwell and Davies
2007). Such shifts were then often sustained for lengthy periods of time –
more than an hour in some cases. On the whole, then, these findings indicate that Intensive Interaction produces fairly dramatic and prolonged
increases in social engagement, and that one does not need to be an experienced practitioner to be aware of them.

It is worth also commenting on the extent to which using Intensive
Interaction intensified the volunteers' sense of connection to the children. All but one of the participants (N=11) remarked spontaneously, at
some point in their reflections, on the ways in which they believed Intensive Interaction had changed their relationships with the children.

> When I tried imitation with Flavius and got such excitement and
> attention from him, it really felt like we were having a conversa-

tion. I found this remarkable, as I had found it difficult to engage with him before. [7]

What we've been introduced to this week is amazing. Everything that we were told did work... I feel like I've been witness to something special and am grateful to have had that opportunity. It will, however, make saying goodbye really hard, but the children's lives will hopefully improve. [4]

It felt really good because before trying imitation it was hard to feel as though I had made a difference, at the end of the day. Whereas when I had used Intensive Interaction, Mircea was having a better time and so was I, because I could see that he was enjoying himself. [5]

It made me feel so delighted to feel that I had broken down a 'barrier' that Serghei puts up as a form of self-defence. [12]

These experiences come despite doubts that the volunteers may have held initially about the use of the technique.

Because Nela was already so friendly, I had my doubts that imitation would have any significant effect on her behaviour. But this turned out not to be true. [1]

I thought that it could be pointless for me to imitate Alina... Nevertheless, I was interested in testing this technique... So I sat down and attempted to imitate her movements and singing. To my surprise, after a few minutes of persistence, Alina was facing me...and her interaction with me was more personal. I have no doubt that the imitation technique I attempted intensified the level of engagement I was able to have with her. [10]

It is obvious that Intensive Interaction had a significant emotional impact on these newly trained practitioners. Not only does this reinforce one of Intensive Interaction theorists' central assertions about the impact of mutual engagement, it also highlights a useful reminder in the development of intervention programmes. Practitioners' motivation and commitment to clients (or children) intensifies once they feel they have established a bond with them.

Discussion

The aim of this project was to extend the use of Intensive Interaction to a new group of people who have previously not had access to it: children with communicative impairments caused by early severe neglect. We hoped to find that Intensive Interaction would increase the level of engagement between children and volunteer carers, even on the basis of very limited training. We believe that the quantitative and qualitative analyses we have carried out provide evidence supporting our expectations.

At a quantitative level, we have been able to show that, on average, our children spent significantly more time engaged in eye-contact with their caregivers during sessions of Intensive Interaction, as compared to standard sessions. Moreover, a high proportion of the group demonstrated this pattern of increased engagement. We interpret these findings as evidence that the children have become more engaged in the interactions with their caregivers – that they have become more willing and able to communicate. The findings relating to physical contact did not show this pattern. The amount of time that children spent touching their partners could not be attributed to the imitative style of responsiveness. While this initially seems to undermine our hypotheses, a more thoughtful examination of the videotapes suggests that our hypothesis was wrong. In the standard sessions, many children were passive and spent much of their time passively sitting close to their caregiver, whereas, in the Intensive Interaction sessions, they became more animated, with several initiating games of chasing tag. While this led to a *decrease* in physical contact, it cannot be said that this was a decrease in engagement, for the children often looked back to make sure that their partner was chasing them. This sense of increased animation can be discerned in the volunteers' comments. Close contact is often taken as an indicator of engagement between mothers and their young babies but, on reflection, this is too simplistic a measure to have chosen for use with these older children.

The qualitative data obtained from the narrative accounts of the volunteers very much confirmed our expectations. In their descriptions of their experiences, these young people make it clear how effective they found Intensive Interaction to be in establishing engagement with the children. It is particularly interesting, and gratifying, to see how often they use the word 'joy' in their accounts. Intensive Interaction helped their relationships with these withdrawn children to become more joyful!

Joy is a difficult variable to define and measure systematically, but it is a word which we hear many people using when we show them our tapes.

One question which needs to be asked is whether Intensive Interaction was of benefit to *all* of the children in the study. Calculating data on the basis of group means does not address this question, while examining the proportion of children showing an increase does. In regard to the findings for eye gaze, the ratio of eight increases to four decreases (in addition to four who showed no change) demonstrates that not all children were benefiting in the same way from Intensive Interaction. The narrative accounts of our volunteer practitioners tend to paint a rosier picture, with *all* of the children being described as having shown some increase in engagement following the introduction of Intensive Interaction into their interactions. These flag important contrasts to investigate in future work, for it would be not be expected that Intensive Interaction would work identically with all children. As Caldwell (2005) emphasises, trainees are learning to speak the individual language of their partner, and the behaviours and abilities of children will differ. It is therefore expected that the form that engagement takes will differ across children; it is inappropriate to assume it will look the same for everyone. One factor which might have a particular influence in the group we were working with here could be the *level* of communicative impairment shown by individual children. Some of our children were beginning to exhibit some (if limited) capacity for linguistic speech, and at least one was known to be an elective mute. It may be that Intensive Interaction works less well in cases where individuals have some speech capacity; indeed, this is what Nadel (2002) would predict. Issues such as this need to be considered in future research.

Another factor which merits further attention concerns practitioner training and skill. In this study our practitioners received a very short training programme before being exhorted to go out and 'try it'. In the light of this minimalist approach we were gratified by the positive results which were achieved, but there is no doubt that our volunteers varied in their susceptibility to these instructions and that the children varied in the challenges with which they presented to volunteers. In Chapter 7, Pete Coia and Angela Jardine Handley describe what they call the OWL-TEA-P cycle of Intensive Interaction. This cycle sees Intensive Interaction as a process of hypothesis testing, with interventions being systematically tried and tested, and only those that 'work' being retained. In the short time period over which our study was conducted it would have been difficult for the volunteer practitioners to problem solve in this way, which implies that even greater increases in engagement might be achieved once the practitioners become more experienced.

In all studies of Intensive Interaction an abiding concern is whether the improvements which are observed can be consolidated so that they last over time. In many of the case studies described by practitioners (Caldwell 2004, 2006; Zeedyk, Caldwell and Davies 2007) the break-throughs in communication between client and therapist are a sufficient end in themselves, and the pleasure that derives from being able to hold some sort of conversation, in the client's own 'language', facilitates the establishment of new relationships between the clients and their care-givers. However, in the case of the Romanian children with whom we were working here it is hoped that the improvements in engagement achieved through the use of Intensive Interaction will lead, in time, to a reduction in quasi-autistic symptoms and the establishment of language skills. In this hope we are encouraged by the experience of Romanian or-phans who were adopted by families in Britain and North America. Many of these children exhibited the symptoms of institutionalised autism when first placed with their adoptive families, but in all cases these symp-toms decreased as the children acclimatised to their new homes (Rutter *et al.* 1999, 2001).

In conclusion, then, we believe that we have been able to demonstrate the efficacy of Intensive Interaction as a means of establishing improved levels of engagement between severely neglected children and their care-givers. This must be seen as only a first step on a journey towards more complete rehabilitation and integration into society. Many 'irrecuperable' children still languish in institutionalised care in the former communist states of Eastern Europe. It is our hope that Intensive Interaction may pro-vide a means of bringing about their rescue.

ACKNOWLEDGEMENTS

Sincere thanks are offered to all the student volunteers who so enthusias-tically participated in this study. Sandu and Alex Micu are commended for their vision in establishing Casa Luminii, as are the charities LIM and MedLink Romania Appeal who have provided funding for the Centre over the last several years. More information on the current operation of the MedLink Appeal (since renamed the Child and Adolescent Support

Team and now operating in other regions of world, in addition to their Romania efforts) can be obtained on www.cast-uk.com.

References

Beebe, B., Jaffe, J., Feldstein, S., Mays, K. and Alson, D. (1985) 'Inter-personal Timing: The Application of an Adult Dialogue Model to Mother–Infant Vocal and Kinetic Interactions.' In T.M. Field and N. Fox (eds) *Social Perception in Infants.* Norwood, NJ: Ablex.

Caldwell, P. (2004) *Crossing the Minefield: Establishing Safe Passage through the Sensory Chaos of Austistic Spectrum Disorder.* Brighton: Pavilion Publishing.

Caldwell, P. (2005) *Creative Conversations: Communicating with People with Profound and Multiple Learning Disabilities.* Brighton: Pavilion Publishing.

Caldwell, P. (2006) *Finding You, Finding Me: Using Intensive Interaction to Get in Touch with People whose Severe Learning Disabilities are Combined with Autism Spectrum Disorder.* London: Jessica Kingsley Publishers.

Chisholm, K. (1998) 'A three-year follow-up of attachment and indiscriminate friendliness in children adopted from Romanian orphanages.' *Child Development 69,* 1092–1106.

Csibra, G. and Gergely, G. (2005) 'Social Learning and Social Cognition: The Case for Pedagogy.' In M.H. Johnson and Y. Munakata (eds) *Processes of Change in Brain and Cognitive Development.* Oxford: Oxford University Press.

Ephraim, G. (1986) *A Brief Introduction to Augmented Mothering.* Radlett: Harperbury Hospital School.

Federici, R.S. (1999) 'Neuropsychological evaluation and rehabilitation of the post institutionalised child.' Presentation at the Conference for Children and Residential Care Stockholm, 3 May 1999. Accessed on 21/02/08 at www.drfederici.com/post_child.htm.

Fisher, L., Ames, E.W., Chisholm, K. and Savoie, L. (1997) 'Problems reported by parents of Romanian orphans adopted to British Coumbia.' *International Journal of Behavioral Development 20,* 67–82.

Garner, P., Hinchcliffe, V. and Sandow, S. (1995) *What Teachers Do: Developments in Special Education.* London: Paul Chapman.

Gloviczki, P.J. (2004) 'Ceausescu's children: The process of democratization and the plight of Romania's orphans.' *Critique: A Worldwide Student Journal of Politics.* Illinois State University, 116–125.

Ingersoll, B. and Gergans, S. (2007) 'The effect of parent-implemented imitation intervention on spontaneous imitation skills in young children with autism.' *Research in Developmental Disabilities 28,* 163–175.

Kaler, S.R. and Freeman, B.J. (1994) 'Analysis of environmental deprivation: Cognitive and social development in Romanian orphans.' *Journal of Child Psychology and Psychiatry 35,* 769–778.

Langton, E.G. (2006) 'Romania's children.' *Psychologist 19,* 412–413.

Meltzoff, A.N. and Gopnik, A. (1993) 'The Role of Imitation in Understanding Persons and Developing Theories of Mind.' In S. Baron-Cohen, H. Tager-Flusberh and D. Cohen (eds) *Understanding Other Minds: Perspectives From Autism.* Oxford: Oxford University Press.

Meltzoff, A.N. and Moore, M.K. (1977) 'Imitation of facial and manual gestures by neonates.' *Science 198*, 75–78.

Morrison, S.J. and Ellwood, A.L. (2000) 'Resiliency in the aftermath of deprivation: A second look at the development of Romanian orphanage children.' *Merrill-Palmer Quarterly 46*, 717–737.

Nadel, J. (2002) 'Imitation and Imitation Recognition: Functional Use in Preverbal Infants and Nonverbal Children with Autism.' In A.N. Meltzoff and W. Prinz (eds) *The Imitative Mind.* Cambridge: Cambridge University Press.

Nadel, J., Revel, A., Andry, P. and Gaussier, P. (2004) 'Toward communication: First imitations in infants, low-functioning children with autism, and robots.' *Interaction Studies 5*, 45–74.

Nind, M. (1996) 'Efficacy of Intensive Interaction: Developing sociability and communication in people with severe and complex learning difficulties using an approach based on care-giver interaction.' *European Journal of Special Needs Education 11*, 48–66.

Nind, M. and Hewett, D. (1994) *Access to Communication.* London: David Fulton Publishers.

Nind, M. and Hewett, D. (2001) *A Practical Guide to Intensive Interaction.* Kidderminster: British Institute of Learning Disabilities.

Nind, M. and Kellett, M. (2002) 'Responding to individuals with severe learning difficulties and stereotyped behaviour: Challenges for an inclusive era.' *European Journal of Special Needs Education 3*, 265–282.

O'Connor, T.G., Bredenkamp, D., Rutter, M. and the English and Romanian Adoptees (ERA) Study Team (2000) 'Attachment disturbances and disorders in children exposed to early severe deprivation.' *Infant Mental Health Journal 20*, 10–29.

O'Neill, M. (2006) 'Imitation as an intervention with children with autistic spectrum disorder and their parents/carers.' PhD thesis, University of Dundee.

O'Neill, M. and Zeedyk, M.S. (2006) 'Spontaneous imitation in the social interactions of young people with developmental delay and their adult carers.' *Infant and Child Development 15*, 283–295.

Rochat, P. (2007) 'Intentional action arises from early reciprocal exchanges.' *Acta Psychologia 124*, 8–25.

Rutter, M. and the English and Romanian Adoptees (ERA) Study Team (1998) 'Developmental catch-up and deficit following adoption after severe global early privation.' *Journal of Child Psychology and Psychiatry 39*, 465–476.

Rutter, M., Andersen-Wood, L., Beckett, C., Bredenkamp, D. *et al.* (1999) 'Quasi-autistic patterns following severe early global privation.' *Journal of Child Psychology and Psychiatry 40*, 537–549.

Rutter, M., Kreppner, J.M., O'Connor, T. and the English and Romanian Adoptees (ERA) Study Team (2001) 'Specificity and heterogeneity in children's responses to profound institutional privation.' *British Journal of Psychiatry 179*, 97–103.

Smyke, A.T., Koga, S.F., Johnson, D.E., Fox, N.A. *et al.* (2007) 'The caregiving context in institution-reared and family-reared infants and toddlers in Romania.' *Journal of Child Psychology and Psychiatry 48*, 210–218.

Sparling, J., Dragomir, C., Ramey, S.L. and Florescu, L. (2005) 'An educational intervention improves developmental progress of young children in a Romanian orphanage.' *Infant Mental Health Journal 26*, 127–142.

Spitz, R. (1945) 'Hospitalism: An inquiry into the genesis of psychiatric conditions in early childhood.' *Psychoanalytic Study of the Child 1*, 53–74.

Stern, D.N. (1985) *The Interpersonal World of the Infant.* New York: Basic Books.

Talbot, M. (1998) 'The disconnected: Attachment theory – the ultimate experiment.' *New York Times,* 24 May. http://query.nytimes.com/gst/fullpage.html?res=940CE1DF1 639F937A15756COA96E958260.

Trevarthen, C. (1978) 'Modes of Perceiving and Modes of Acting.' In H.L. Pick and E. Saltzman (eds) *Modes of Perceiving and Processing Information.* Cambridge University Press: Cambridge.

Van den Tillart, B. (2000) 'Encouraging reciprocity in interaction with deafblind people and their partners.' *Deafblind Review 25*, 6–8.

Watson, J. and Fisher, A. (1997) 'Evaluating the effectiveness of Intensive Interaction teaching with pupils with profound and complex learning difficulties.' *British Journal of Special Education 24*, 80–87.

Zeedyk, M.S. (2006) 'From intersubjectivity to subjectivity: The transformative roles of emotional intimacy and imitation.' *Infant and Child Development 15*, 321–344.

Zeedyk, M.S., Caldwell, P. and Davies, C.E. (in press) 'How rapidly does Intensive Interaction promote social engagement for adults with profound learning disabilities and communicative impairments?' *European Journal of Special Needs Education.*

Zeedyk, M.S., Davies, C.E., Parry, S. and Caldwell, P. (in press) 'Fostering social engagement in Romanian children with communicative impairments: The experiences of newly trained practitioners of Intensive Interaction.' *British Journal of Learning Disabilities.*

CHAPTER 7

DEVELOPING RELATIONSHIPS WITH PEOPLE WITH PROFOUND LEARNING DISABILITIES THROUGH INTENSIVE INTERACTIONS

Pete Coia and Angela Jardine Handley

Sarah and Daniel looked different from the others, that much was obvious to Michael when he entered the room. Everyone else was sitting alone: some people were rocking, some sleeping, others were staring into space. Sarah and Daniel were sitting together, facing each other. Michael thought they looked like they were talking about something.

As Michael got closer to Sarah and Daniel, he noticed that they weren't making a sound. He couldn't see exactly what they were doing, but he thought they may be taking something apart together, or trying to fix something that was awkward to hold.

Sarah and Daniel were so engrossed in what they were doing, that Michael was able to sit down, apparently unnoticed, close beside them. From here Michael could see clearly what they were doing. Sitting silently, Sarah and Daniel were touching each others' hands. First one would do something, and then the other would do something a bit different, and so on. Michael knew that Sarah and Daniel were having a conversation and one which looked quite complicated.

Michael didn't know what to do next. He couldn't join in because he didn't understand exactly how to and he was beginning to feel uncomfortable watching Sarah and Daniel: as if somehow he was intruding on their private, even intimate, moment together.

As he quietly got up to leave, it struck Michael that you couldn't tell from observing them together whether it was Sarah or Daniel who had the labels 'profound learning disability', 'autism' or 'professional'.

Then, a darker thought entered Michael's mind. Maybe that is why some people think Intensive Interaction is difficult or inappropriate.

Intensive Interaction is an approach to communicating with people with learning disabilities. As other chapters in this volume show, it is also gaining attention in other areas, including autism, sensory impairment, and dementia (for example, see Chapters 4, 5, 6, 8 and 11). For some people, using Intensive Interaction is an intuitive process which requires little, if any, cognitive effort. For others, however, it is useful to rely on an explicit conceptual model of Intensive Interaction. Our key aim in writing this chapter is to provide such a model: to explain Intensive Interaction from our perspective.

As clinical practitioners we have extensive experience of working with a wide range of people with learning disabilities and their carers. Currently we provide our services to adults with learning disabilities as part of an NHS Specialist Assessment and Treatment service. Throughout our years of clinical practice we have each used Intensive Interaction, and over the past ten years have developed the conceptual model of Intensive Interaction described here to guide others in its use. Our chapter is therefore written from our perspectives both as clinicians and providers of Intensive Interaction training.

The model we use originates in observations of 'typical' communication and therefore applies to communication between human beings in general. However, we have focused within the chapter on the use of the model as a way of understanding Intensive Interaction and therefore supporting communication between adults with profound learning disabilities and their carers. We hope our model will be particularly useful to those who find Intensive Interaction isn't always an effortless and intuitive process, those who, just like us, get 'stuck' sometimes.

The description at the beginning of the chapter was of a genuine intensive interaction (except that the people's names have been changed). It captures a number of important and observable characteristics of an intensive interaction, which we will now highlight and discuss using our model.

A model of Intensive Interaction

Intensive Interaction is one way of building a relationship between two people. Usually, one person is a professional, with a culturally typical communication style. The other person usually has an unusual, or unique, communication style and a label such as 'severe learning disability', 'profound and multiple learning disability' and/or 'autism'.

A relationship is usually built through the use of appropriate and meaningful communication. Between 'normal' adults this conversation takes the form of various types of conversations.

We use a model of a 'typical' conversation, the good verbal conversations *we* like to have, as a way of understanding and modelling an '-intensive interaction'. In reality, a 'typical' conversation, like all communication, can be extremely complicated but we are going to deliberately simplify things without, we hope, oversimplifying them.

A TYPICAL CONVERSATION

Typical conversations generally have two communication partners and two roles. The roles are speaker and listener. Each communication partner takes their turn in each role. So, while one person speaks the other listens, and vice versa, throughout the conversation – although not waiting for your turn can be a problem for some people sometimes!

In typical conversations both people will be using words, sounds and gestures in similar ways, and so will understand each other. I know what you mean because the sounds you make when you speak are the same as the ones I make when I speak. For example, when you say 'hello' you make the same sounds that I make when I say 'hello', therefore, when you say 'hello' you must mean what I mean when I say 'hello'.

A SHARED CULTURAL LIBRARY

This shared use of words, sounds and gestures, and their meanings, can be conceptualised as a *shared cultural library*. In the UK this shared cultural library contains the non-verbal sounds, signs and rules used in the *English language*. For example, these rules govern whom we talk to, how we talk to them, what topics are acceptable in particular conversations, how close you are to the person you are talking to and how loudly to speak. This cultural library is developed by exposure to and understanding of a particular culture.

While some of this shared cultural library is written down, such as the sound–word–meaning links found in a dictionary, most of it is only contained within the minds of the people in that cultural community. Most typical adults, within that community, will have enough grasp of their shared cultural library to understand each other extremely well. For example, within a conversation by members of the same cultural community, very subtle shades of emotion and meaning can be effectively communicated.

A UNIQUE SUB-CULTURAL LIBRARY

Within a particular conversation, what the speaker is currently saying, and what the listener understands as a result, is influenced by what has already been communicated between them – both within that conversation and their previous conversations. In this sense, any conversation between two people reflects their entire conversational history. For example, what we talk about with people we know well is different from what we talk about in our first conversation with someone. Furthermore, our current conversations add to, and change, our expanding conversational history.

This expanding conversational history, within a particular relationship, is subject to a kind of evolution. Topics and rules which were part of previously successful conversations, but which are not part of the general cultural library, are incorporated into a *sub-cultural library* that is unique to that relationship. For example, the authors of this article do not talk to anyone else about Intensive Interaction in the way they talk to each other!

A NON-CONVERSATION

What happens if two people try to have a conversation but don't share a cultural library? If there is little, or no, overlap between the two individuals' cultural libraries, each person may not understand what the other is saying, or even recognise that the other person is trying to say something. Each person may tell him- or herself that the other has a serious communication problem, or simply lacks the ability to communicate at all. Therefore, a 'non-conversation' occurs.

Unlike good conversations, these non-conversations are typically emotionally difficult. We may, for example, feel frustrated, disappointed, or useless if we can't find a way of communicating, despite our motivation to do so. Unsurprisingly, we may try to avoid feeling these types of unpleasant emotions by simply avoiding the person who we believe makes us feel them. Unfortunately, this type of avoidance makes the communication problem permanent! In contrast, if there is enough motivation, each person may try to learn the other's language. In practice, one person may find this easier than the other, particularly if one person is more able, and has more experience at learning other languages.

THE CULTURAL LIBRARIES OF PEOPLE WITH LEARNING DISABILITIES

Sadly, these non-conversations often describe the relationship between professionals and people with learning disabilities and/or autism. Within a professional relationship between a typical adult and a person with a different communication style, the typical English cultural library is not available. By definition, the person with a different communication style isn't using it.

Even when exposed to our cultural library, people with learning disabilities and/or autism don't experience and understand it in the way that we typically do. In this sense, they don't really become an integral part of our culture. As a result people with a learning disability and/or autism develop their own, and often unique, cultural library derived from their own specific, and often very different, experiences.

As different people with learning disabilities and/or autism have different histories, it is not surprising that there is no standard 'learning disability/autistic cultural library' that we can learn and use with everyone who has these labels.

Intensive Interaction: The core task

Generally, communication-based interventions for people with learning disabilities and/or autism focus on teaching individuals our English shared cultural library, or some variation of it. The Intensive Interaction practice we are describing here does the exact *opposite*.

The core task within Intensive Interaction is for the professional to learn the other person's unique cultural library, his or her unique non-verbal 'language' and its 'rules'.

It is this unique cultural library which can be used by both the professional and person who has learning disabilities and/or autism to have conversations and to build their relationship. Additionally, together they may be able to develop a more extensive sub-cultural library within their ongoing relationship, based on what they learn about each other and their shared experience.

Importantly, any developing sub-cultural library, within an Intensive Interaction based relationship, may never achieve the highly developed nature of the more usual 'English' cultural library. Some things may never be expressible using the developing sub-cultural library of the relationship. For example, the person with a learning disability and/or autism may never be able to communicate with us about yesterday's TV news.

THE IMPORTANCE OF TALKING TO YOURSELF

Everyone 'talks' to themselves, and everyone does it in a way that they understand, that is meaningful to them. This is simply having a 'conversation' with yourself. Just as with the development of a typical conversational history between two people, meaningless topics fall out of the repertoire of our conversations with ourselves: we develop our own unique cultural library.

How people talk to themselves is important for our Intensive Interaction practice, because people with learning disabilities and/or autism 'talk' to themselves too. If we recognise and understand the unique cultural library that the person with a learning disability and/or autism is using with him- or herself, we can use it to have a conversation with that person.

To discover how people talk to themselves we use three key models:

- the OWL-TEA-P cycle

- the ABCS of meaning

- the comfort zones.

We will outline these models, and then apply them to Sarah and Daniel's intensive interaction described at the beginning of this chapter.

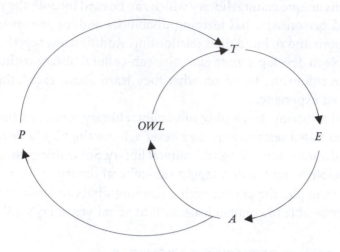

Figure 7.1: OWL: Observe, Wait, Listen

THE OWL-TEA-P CYCLE

The OWL-TEA-P cycle is an explicit reflective practice model. Each letter is one step in a repeating pattern of practice steps – we usually start with the OWL step and then go through all the other steps. We use a visual representation of this model (see Figure 7.1).

OWL: Observe, Wait, Listen

An observation is something you can sense directly. Usually, observations are what you can see and hear or sometimes what you can touch and smell. For example, a description of the way someone moves his or her body is an observation: 'Alan raised his arm, with his fingers curled over into his palm.' If different people are observing the same thing, they should have the same observations.

T: Theory (translation)

The observer uses a theory to translate (change) his or her observations into explanations. This happens sub-consciously, and very fast, often resulting in two specific problems.

First, people often do not realise that this theory stage is occurring. This means that when asked for a description of behaviour (observations), they often provide explanations instead without realising that they have done so. For example when asked to describe Alan's behaviour, staff said 'Alan was being aggressive' (explanation) rather than 'Alan raised his arm, with his fingers curled into his palm' (observation).

Second, people are usually unaware of the theory they are using, and that their theory has come from their own cultural library. This is one reason why different observers come up with different explanations, even if they have observed the same events. For example, two workers may have the same observation that 'Alan raised his arm, with his fingers curled over into his palm.' Nonetheless, while one of them explains this observation as 'Alan was being aggressive' the other explains it as 'that's how Alan says hello'.

E: Explanation

An explanation is a statement about what particular observations mean, such as why behaviour occurred. For example, 'Alan was being aggressive' is an explanation of the observation 'Alan raised his arm, with his fingers curled over into his palm.' Different people may have different explanations for the same observations.

A: Action

An action is what the observer, or conversational partner, does in response, based on his or her explanation. For example, the worker with the aggression explanation restrained Alan. Clearly, if a worker has a different explanation, such as 'this is Alan saying "hello"', he or she may take a different action, such as say 'hello' back to Alan.

P: Prediction

A prediction is what the person believes will happen as a result of the action(s). For example, when Alan was restrained, the worker predicted that he would not be hit or hurt by Alan.

HOW PEOPLE TALK TO THEMSELVES AND THE OWL-TEA-P CYCLE

Observing and listening (OWLing) individuals talking to themselves provides evidence about the unique cultural library they use with themselves. For example, OWLing people with learning disabilities and/or autism may reveal how they touch or move parts of themselves or the sounds they simultaneously make and hear. In contrast, listening to 'typical' people talking to themselves out loud reveals what verbal language they are using – in the UK, this is often English.

Creating a conversation, however, is not as straightforward as 'you are using particular sounds or movements so I will too'. As in a typical verbal conversation, there is more to it than simply repeating the same words that you have just heard! Nonetheless, if you speak non-verbally to a non-verbal person, using that person's type of non-verbal *words* and *rules*, you will be using his or her cultural library. Unsurprisingly, the person is then more likely to understand you and, importantly for interaction, respond to you.

ABCS AND COMFORT ZONES: THE BIG T IN THE OWL-TEA-P CYCLE

The 'ABCS of meaning' and 'comfort zones' provide an overall theory to translate our observations into explanations.

THE ABCS OF MEANING

What we term the 'ABCS of meaning' is our attempt to make explicit some of the different types of meaning that statements and actions can have. For example, when you hear the words 'the train is late', they will have affective (A), behavioural (B), cognitive (C) and sensory (S) meanings for you.

The cognitive meaning (C) is the intellectual information in your mind. For example, 'the time on the timetable is different from the time that the train will arrive'. The affective meaning (A) is how you feel emotionally. For example, you may have been feeling bored while waiting for the train but now feel very sad, angry or even happy. Whether you are now sad, angry or happy depends upon other cognitive meanings, such as whether the train being late means you miss something you were dreading going to, or something you really wanted to attend.

The behavioural meaning (B) is, unsurprisingly, how you behave. For example, you may have been sitting reading the newspaper before you discovered that the 'train is late', but now you are pacing up and down, rubbing your chin, breathing more quickly, and talking to yourself!

The sensory meaning (S) is the physical sensations you experience. For example, while you were sitting down reading the newspaper, you may not have been aware of any particular physical sensations, or those that you were aware of seemed comfortable. Now that you are sad or angry, and pacing up and down, you may be aware of a physical sensation of tenseness or a feeling of being hot and thirsty.

COMFORT ZONES

Comfort zones are where we are comfortable – as you can easily guess, when we are outside our comfort zones we are uncomfortable, even distressed. Importantly, for each aspect of meaning, affective (A), behavioural (B), cognitive (C) or sensory (S), there is a corresponding comfort zone.

We'll start with the sensory comfort zone – this is the range of physical sensations with which we feel comfortable. For example, in relation to temperature, when we feel too hot or too cold we feel physically uncomfortable and are outside of our sensory comfort zone.

A common cause of people being pushed out of their cognitive comfort zone is when they are being given too much information, typically in words. For example, this happens when too many people are speaking to you, or asking you to do too many things at the same time, or you don't understand the information you are being given because it is not based on your cultural library. People are often pushed out of their behavioural comfort zone when they are trying to do too many things at once or when they don't have enough to do.

When people have emotional feelings that they don't want to have, and don't feel comfortable with, they are outside of their affective comfort zone. For example, this can occur when we like people we believe we shouldn't like, or when we dislike people that we should like.

While the affective and sensory zones may seem the most familiar, the cognitive and behavioural comfort zones are equally important in everyday life.

There are three important points to consider about comfort zones.

First, the limits of each of the comfort zones (A, B, C and S) are different for each person. Furthermore, a particular person's limits can change over time and in different situations.

Second, the different comfort zones are all interconnected. If you change your position on one comfort zone, for better or worse, you will automatically change your position on all of the other ones. For example, having a bath when you feel physically tense is physically relaxing – it is a sensory action, but it will also make you feel better emotionally, while also changing your thoughts (cognitions) and behaviour.

Third, it is usually much easier to accidentally, or even deliberately, push someone with a learning disability and/or autism out of his or her comfort zones. For example, relative to a typical person, having a learning disability and/or autism usually means that you are:

- able to cope with less information, and need that information delivered at a slower pace, within your own unique cultural library

- often told what to do and not to do

- often required to behave in ways that you find difficult, unpleasant or even impossible.

GETTING BACK IN TO YOUR COMFORT ZONES

So, what do people do when they are outside of their comfort zones? Usually, they do something to get themselves back into their comfort zones, if they can and if they know how to.

For example, if you are outside your sensory comfort zone, by being too hot or cold, you can change your temperature by adjusting the heating or the amount of clothes you are wearing. Similarly, if you are outside your affective (emotional) comfort zone, let's say you are feeling unhappy, you might talk to someone who cares a lot about you, or get a hug from him or her, and so feel better emotionally. You may even do something by yourself, such as talk to yourself, or have a nice warm bath with a glass of fine wine alongside a good book!

The key point is that when *you* are outside of your comfort zones you do something, with someone else or by yourself, which positively influences your ABCS, so that you get back into your comfort zones. Importantly, what one person does to get back into, or stay in, his or her comfort zones can be different from the next person, irrespective of whether the people concerned have, or don't have, a learning disability and/or autism. We call the things individuals do to regain, or remain within, their comfort zones 'comfort behaviours'.

ABCS, COMFORT ZONES AND INTENSIVE INTERACTION

In relation to Intensive Interaction, we believe three things are particularly important when considering the ABCS of meaning and comfort zones for people with learning disabilities and/or autism.

First, people with learning disabilities and/or autism are often very experienced at engaging in their comfort behaviours on their own. These behaviours often become the person's mannerisms. When these comfort behaviours are noticed by professionals, these are sometimes seen as a problem and attract labels like 'stereotyped' or 'repetitive' behaviours.

Second, the comfort that people with learning disabilities and/or autism give themselves is often (but not always) sensory in nature. Put another way, they use behaviours, which are often sensory in nature, to talk to themselves: to keep themselves in, or return themselves to, their comfort zones.

Third, if we are going to talk to people with severe or profound learning disabilities and/or autism, then learning to use the parts of their unique cultural library that are embedded in their comfort behaviours seems like a good place to begin. In our Intensive Interaction practice, it is these comfort behaviours that we consider to be the individuals talking to themselves, in the most helpful way they are aware of.

The OWL-TEA-P Cycle and Intensive Interaction in practice: An example

In this section, we will use the models we have outlined to think about Daniel and Sarah's conversation: their intensive interaction.

OWLINGS

Sarah had made detailed observations of Daniel, over a number of days. For example, Sarah had observed that Daniel was almost always alone, sitting in his chair. He had a number of toys next to him on a table, including a musical telephone, several story and musical books, and two soft toys. Staff reported that Daniel often played with these toys. Staff also offered the explanation that Daniel really liked listening to the music these toys made. However, Sarah noticed that Daniel *played* with the toys even when the batteries had run out and they failed to make any musical noises.

Looking closely, Sarah also noticed that Daniel did a number of things with the different toys. He held them in his hands so that they touched his palms. He squeezed and released them. He moved or rubbed them between his fingers. He pressed them with his fingertips. When Daniel touched the toys, he usually did so using a particular, and quite slow, rhythm.

THEORY AND EXPLANATIONS

Sarah used the ABCS of meaning and comfort zones theory to translate her observations into explanations. For example, Sarah had observed that the amount of toy touching Daniel did increased, as did the rhythm of his touching, when there were more people and more noise in his immediate environment. Sarah's explanation was that Daniel's toy touching was a comfort behaviour. This behaviour got him back into his comfort zones, which he had been pushed out of by the increase in activity and noise around him.

Sarah also had a number of possible explanations about why the toy touching was an effective comfort behaviour. For example, she thought that Daniel's touching could be focused on the sensory qualities of touching the toys (the 'S' of the ABCS of meaning). Sarah had also considered a cognitive/affective explanation for Daniel's touching behaviours – control. In this sense, Sarah thought that Daniel's rhythmical and repetitive toy touching may have given him the feeling of control, and cognitive certainty of knowing what will happen next.

Sarah knew that if the correct meaning of Daniel's comfort behaviours was primarily sensory, rather than to do with control, then other ways of supplying that sensory feedback could become part of his unique cultural library. Consequently, using similar forms of sensory feedback should capture Daniel's attention and become an effective way of having a non-verbal conversation with him. In contrast, if it was control that Daniel wanted, then such sensory based actions would probably be ineffective, as Daniel might experience them as interfering and thus reducing his level of control.

Sarah decided to initially pursue her sensory explanation – actually she had a list of several possible sensory explanations. In compiling her list, Sarah had asked herself a number of questions, including:

- What is it about the feel of the toys that Daniel finds calming?

- Is it the rhythm of the touching or the pressure that he gets through his skin?

- Does he seem to get the same feedback from each of the toys or is his experience with each toy different – is he using different toys to have different conversations with himself?

Sarah also tried to replicate for herself exactly what she had seen Daniel doing with each of the toys to try to experience directly the sensory feedback he might be getting from his toys.

In the end, Sarah decided to take actions based on two possible sensory explanations of the way that Daniel was 'talking' to himself – he could be primarily interested in the rhythm or the pressure of the touch, or both.

ACTIONS

To test her explanations, Sarah knew she had to take actions one at a time, so that she could understand which, if any, had an effect on Daniel. She wanted to take an action which could develop into an interaction; an action that would have the same, or better, effect on Daniel than the comfort behaviour he was using to talk to himself.

Sarah's first action was tried to test her rhythm explanation. She waited until Daniel was engaged in the touching behaviours and tapped him on his forearm using the same rhythm that he was using to squeeze his toy.

PREDICTIONS

Sarah recognised that testing her explanations was about predicting what would happen as a result of her actions. She knew that if her explanations were wrong then her predictions would also be wrong – her predictions would not match her next set of observations.

Sarah chose to tap Daniel's forearm because of her prediction that if it was the rhythm that Daniel was interested in, then he would be interested in that rhythm even if he wasn't experiencing it through his hands. If it wasn't the rhythm then he was unlikely to be interested in it.

When Sarah tapped Daniel's arm she had predicted that Daniel would stop rhythmically squeezing the toy he was holding, because her rhythm would be more interesting for Daniel.

Once Sarah had rhythmically tapped Daniel she waited; he didn't stop squeezing his toy. Sarah tried this a few times, just in case Daniel was unaware of her actions, but Daniel didn't stop squeezing his toy: Sarah's predictions had been wrong. This made her think that her rhythm explanation was wrong.

GOING AROUND THE OWL-TEA-P CYCLE

Sarah repeated her tapping. She wasn't ready to give up on her rhythm explanation just yet. Sarah thought 'maybe it is the rhythm, but I am giving Daniel the rhythm in the wrong place'. So, Sarah rhythmically tapped Daniel a few more times but in different places: she tapped his knee and his shoulder, repeating the tapping several times in each place.

Sarah again predicted that Daniel would stop squeezing his toy. Daniel didn't stop squeezing his toy: Sarah's predictions were wrong again!

Sarah finally gave up on her rhythm explanation. She knew that it did not matter that her rhythm explanation had been wrong. She knew that this was simply part of the process of testing out her explanations. Anyway, she had observed that when she was tapping Daniel his squeezing behaviour had not increased – this pleased her because her explanation of this was that she had not increased Daniel's discomfort with her tapping.

Sarah then tested her pressure explanation. Daniel was holding a teddy bear leg in his hand and squeezing it gently. Sarah put her hand into Daniel's other hand, and squeezed gently, trying to give Daniel the same pressure that he was getting from squeezing the bear. Then she waited.

Sarah had predicted, again, that Daniel would stop squeezing his bear – and this time she was right! Daniel had stopped squeezing his bear. Sarah was beginning to think that her pressure explanation was right, but knew she had to test it out further. So, Sarah continued to gently squeeze Daniel's hand, and then wait. Daniel stopped squeezing his bear again. Sarah and Daniel had managed to say 'hello'.

Saying 'hello' to each other in this way eventually developed into some quite complex conversations using hand pressure. Sarah was beginning to use Daniel's unique cultural library well enough that Daniel had discarded his bear (and other toys) when Sarah was around, so that he could talk to her using both of his hands. It was one of these hand conversations, an 'intensive interaction', that Michael had witnessed when he observed them both.

Importantly Sarah, and Daniel, had been round the OWL-TEA-P cycle a few times before they began to find a way to interact with each other. Fortunately for both them, they were both willing and able to do so.

A summary

We see Intensive Interaction as a non-verbal conversation. In order to develop these conversations we recognise that people with learning disabilities and/or autism do not share our 'English' cultural library. Instead they have a different and often unique cultural library, including a language of their own that they use to talk to themselves. This language is not word based, and is often sensory in nature. The core task in communicating with people with learning disabilities and/or autism is to learn and use their unique cultural library.

In order to discover this unique cultural library we use a reflective practice model called the OWL-TEA-P cycle. We think that if the person is doing something with him- or herself, that person will recognise, understand, and value the meaning of it. So our first task is to observe exactly what the person is doing.

Using the overall theory of the ABCS of meaning and comfort zones, we develop a list of possible explanations for our observations of the other person's behaviour – a list of what that particular behaviour might mean for that individual.

In testing out our explanations, the actions we take are trying to capture and provide the meaning of the other person's behaviour within something that we do. Importantly, we make predictions about the outcome of our actions before we take them.

If our explanations are incorrect we expect our predictions will not match our next set of observations – and that an interaction is unlikely to develop. If our explanations are correct, more or less, then our predictions usually match our next set of observations, and interaction often develops.

Therefore, in testing out our explanations we go around, and around, the OWL-TEA-P cycle until our predictions match our next set of observations. When this happens, we have usually understood enough of the meaning of the other person's behaviour to at least say 'hello' using his or her unique cultural library.

Importantly, in getting this far, we have typically made a number of mistakes. That is, we have taken actions which did not result in our predicted outcomes. The OWL-TEA-P cycle gives us a way to learn from these mistakes, and to keep going until we get it right.

Over time, as with any typical relationship, a unique sub-cultural library containing a repertoire of intensive interactions (non-verbal conversations) will develop. Topics and rules that don't work will drop out of the repertoire whilst topics and rules that work will remain. This unique sub-cultural library may develop and become more varied and rich over time, as it did with Sarah and Daniel.

Although this all sounds very straightforward, we recognise that there can be many challenges on the journey to learning another person's language, particularly one that is so culturally different from our own. An obvious practical difficulty is that this process can require an investment of time and emotions from the practitioner which he or she is not always able, or willing, to make.

In our view, using the OWL-TEA-P cycle is not always necessary but it can be very helpful at times. When one begins to use the OWL-TEA-P cycle, it is used as a conscious and deliberate strategy, an explicit intellectual tool to guide practice. At this early stage, using the cycle can feel very deliberate, slow, and like hard work. With enough practice however, you can use the OWL-TEA-P cycle automatically, and without any apparent conscious effort. At this more advanced stage, using the cycle feels just like using intuition!

As professionals who work with people with learning disabilities and/or autism, and their staff, on a daily basis, we believe that you can't overstate the importance of communication. Everyone communicates in some way, and everybody simply needs to. Without communication, relationships aren't possible – without relationships the very essence of what makes life valuable drains away. In this sense, we feel that Intensive Interaction, or any approach that delivers the same outcomes – good conversations and relationships – is simply a necessary part of everyday living for all of us, including people with learning disabilities and/or autism and the staff who interact with them.

CHAPTER 8

A NEW APPROACH TO COMMUNICATING WITH PEOPLE WITH ADVANCED DEMENTIA: A CASE STUDY OF ADAPTIVE INTERACTION

Maggie P. Ellis and Arlene J. Astell

We are two psychologists who work with people who have a diagnosis of dementia, a progressive, deteriorating condition, which typically affects older people and impacts on all aspects of functioning. Between us we have 25 years of experience working in this field and both have a particular interest in the impact of dementia on communication and the effect this has on relationships between people with dementia and caregivers.

In this chapter we report our first attempt to explore an approach to communication based on Intensive Interaction (II) with an individual in the very advanced stages of dementia. Unlike people with profound learning disabilities or severe autism, for whom II opens up channels of communication for the first time, people with dementia have previously been healthy individuals who communicated through speech. The communication barriers they experience arise from a progressive loss of speech coupled with severe cognitive problems.

In this case study we work with Edie, who is an 81-year-old lady living in a nursing home whose dementia has progressed to the stage where she can no longer speak. We use principles from Intensive Interaction to explore Edie's communication repertoire in an attempt to 'learn her language', now that she no longer has speech. We find that Edie retains an urge to communicate with another person and has a range of behaviours that make up her language. We describe two interactions — one speech-based conversation and the other using the principles of Intensive Interaction – that took place between Edie and one of us (ME) and the outcomes of those interactions.

The findings suggest that an approach to communication based on II has something to offer people with advanced dementia who can no longer speak. However, this population has severe memory problems, which means that no assumptions can be made about building up a repertoire of communication from session to session. Instead, communication partners must approach each interaction with people with advanced dementia as a unique encounter and adapt their behaviour anew each time. We term this approach Adaptive Interaction. In this case study we make no assumptions that Edie will subsequently remember the interaction or the exchange of communication behaviours.

Dementia

Dementia is an illness that involves progressive global decline in all aspects of functioning. Memory is usually affected early in the course of the illness, although all aspects of cognition, including speech, problem solving, perception, decision-making and functional abilities are affected over time (Raia 1999). The symptoms of dementia impede people's ability to participate in most daily activities, not least of which is communication and participation in social interactions.

The majority of people who develop dementia are over 65 and as the illness develops they experience progressive social isolation (Abad 2002). This is a result not only of their increasingly impaired communication skills but also arises as a consequence of those around them making fewer attempts to communicate. By the time dementia reaches the later stages, people with a diagnosis may appear to be completely unreachable, which results in those who care for them no longer attempting to engage them in interactions.

Communication in advanced dementia

The communication problems experienced by people with advanced dementia clearly have a huge impact both on them and on those who care for them. For families, communication difficulties put a major strain on maintaining relationships with the person with dementia, whereas care staff face the challenge of establishing relationships with people whose communication skills are already severely compromised when they first meet. As such, communication and social interactions are extremely difficult and may cease altogether except in pursuance of basic activities of daily living (Bowie and Mountain 1993). This situation is clearly unsatisfying both for people with dementia and for those who care for them.

Improving interpersonal communication in this situation could improve the job satisfaction of care staff and the quality of life of people with dementia (Woods 1999). The challenge is how to facilitate communication when people with dementia have little or no speech and may only make sounds or repeat isolated words or movements. It is argued, however, that even at this advanced stage people retain many identifiable communication skills (Orange and Purves 1996) and demonstrate a continued urge to communicate and interact with others (Ellis and Astell 2004). These retained behaviours could form the basis of an intervention designed specifically for individuals with advanced dementia that has the potential to enhance their lives and the lives of those who care for them.

Intensive Interaction

Intensive Interaction is an approach to interacting with people with severe communication problems that was developed in the 1980s for people with profound learning disabilities. The focus of II is on regular non-verbal and subvocal exchanges with little or no involvement of speech between two people, one of whom experiences difficulty communicating with others. The quality of the interaction is all important in II, and there is no emphasis on task performance or achieving specific outcomes (Nind 1999). The key to II is that the behaviour of the nonverbal participant is viewed as intentionally communicative.

The basic principles of II reflect the essential communicative processes that occur early in life between caregivers and infants (Nind 1999). Although the structure and the linguistic contents of these early exchanges are non-verbal, few people would argue that they are without meaning or emotion (Papoušek 1995; cited in Duffy 1999). Furthermore, Nind (1999) asserted that this similarity in approaches does not mean that people with learning disabilities or, by extension, other severe communication impairments, should be regarded or treated as if they were infants.

Intensive Interaction commences with professionals or caregivers becoming familiar with the person they want to communicate with and the types of interactions that this person might engage in. This initial 'connection' is then developed into a set of spontaneous interactive 'games' that are based on the behaviour of the person with communication impairment. For example, a sound or action he makes, such as banging on the table, might be reflected back by his partner, either directly or with some variation in the rhythm. The professional or caregiver responds contingently to her partner's behaviours to continuously expand the interactions between them and support her partner to take a more active role in communication.

As II has developed over the years, different aspects of the basic approach have been emphasised. Hewett (1996) and Nind (1999), for example, both consider the focus of II to be on teaching the 'pre-speech fundamentals' of communication. These fundamentals include turn taking, shared attention and eye gaze, which are developed together by the two communication partners (Nind 1999). In this approach the professional or caregiver is termed the 'teacher' and the communication-impaired partner the 'learner'. The teacher constantly modifies her own interpersonal behaviours such as body language, eye gaze, vocalisations and facial expressions in order to make them as engaging and as meaningful as possible to their communication-impaired partner. It is important for teachers to be attentive to their partner's behaviour, to create pauses in the interaction and to be open to joining in with rhythms and sounds their partner may make. This may include imitation of certain elements of the communication-impaired partner's behaviour and vocalisations.

In Caldwell's (2005; Caldwell and Horwood 2007) version of II, imitation is the starting point: 'a way of capturing attention, a door to enter the inner world of our partners' (see Chapter 11). Caldwell's' approach to II emphasises exploring the sensory experience of people with profound communication difficulties and attempting to 'learn their language' (Caldwell and Horwood 2007). One key outcome of this approach is providing a way for people typically regarded as outside the social world to express themselves. This is commonly seen in shifts from solitary self-stimulatory behaviour, such as biting or head banging, to engagement in shared activity. By responding in ways that are familiar to the person with severe communication difficulties, i.e. initially imitating and then developing them into a shared 'language', it is possible to build and sustain close relationships without speech.

Studies using II typically employ video-recording to measure developments in communicative responses (e.g. Kellett 2000, 2003; Nind 1996). For example, Nind (1996) examined engaged social interaction, smiling, eye-contact and looking at the communication partner's face. The efficacy of II in increasing the occurrence of such social behaviours in people with severe learning disabilities has been demonstrated in numerous studies (e.g. Samuel and Maggs 1998; Stothard 1998; Watson and Fisher 1997). Additionally, several government bodies have noted other benefits of II, including improved quality of life (DfES 2001a, 2001b; Ofsted 1996/1997, 2000).

Intensive Interaction for advanced dementia

Such benefits and positive effects on communication are clearly very desirable for people with advanced dementia, who are frequently excluded from the social world. Intensive Interaction appears to have great potential for improving communication between people with advanced dementia and those who care for them. To investigate the usefulness of II for facilitating communication with people with advanced dementia we conducted a single case study. We were guided by principles from both of the variants of II discussed above. Caldwell's (2005; Caldwell and Horwood 2007) approach to II with its focus on matched responsiveness and non-verbal behaviour was felt to be best suited to exploiting any retained communication behaviours of people with advanced dementia who no longer have speech. However, Hewett and Nind's (1998) work, which focuses on the pre-speech fundamentals of communication, can be seen as providing a framework for identifying retained communication behaviours. In this case study we attempt to 'learn the language' of a person with advanced dementia and explore the potential for engaging her in meaningful, shared activity.

Case study: Edie

Edie is an 81-year-old lady who has dementia that has reached a very advanced stage. She started to lose speech some years ago but coped initially with everyday tasks such as shopping by writing a list and giving it to an assistant. Later on in her illness Edie began to engage in less functional activity, such as going out to look for her daughter at her place of work in the middle of the night. She eventually became unable to look after herself at home and was admitted to a local care home. Five years on Edie has no speech at all and is unable to walk. She spends most of the day in bed or in front of the television in the residents' lounge. She receives regular visits from her daughter.

Ethical approval for the study was received from the Multicentre Research Ethics Committee (MREC) designated to consider research proposals covered by Section 51 (3) (f) of the Adults with Incapacity (Scotland) Act 2000. In accordance with this legislation, consent for Edie to participate was sought from her nearest family member, her daughter. The ethical approval included video-recording the interactions with Edie and her daughter also consented to this.

LEARNING EDIE'S LANGUAGE

Stage 1: Current communication context

The first step in learning Edie's language was to explore her current communication context. This involved spending two days in the care home observing the everyday activities and communication that took place. Additional information was collected from the manager of the care home and some of the staff. This highlighted that the team responsible for providing Edie's care found it difficult to communicate with her and engage her in activities of daily living such as eating, bathing and toileting.

Edie's daughter was also interviewed as part of understanding her current communication context. Her daughter identified a number of behaviours that she felt had communicative value for Edie, including a high-pitched sound, sucking and chewing her thumb and laughing.

Stage 2: Baseline interaction

The next step in learning Edie's language was to collect baseline data on Edie's communication behaviour. For this we devised a ten-minute session where one of us (ME) went into Edie's room to conduct a spoken conversation consisting of the sort of questions typically asked in day-to-day interactions observed in the care home. These included: 'Did you enjoy your meal?', 'Did you have a lie in this morning?' and 'Have you seen the weather outside today?' Each of these closed questions would be followed by a 20-second pause to give Edie the best possible opportunity to respond in some way, for example by nodding or shaking her head.

Stage 3: Intensive Interaction

Step three of learning Edie's language was to attempt to communicate with her using her own behaviours as the basis of the interaction (Caldwell 2005; Caldwell and Horwood 2007). For this we decided to again allow ten minutes for the same investigator (ME) to go into Edie's room to conduct a session where she would attend to and imitate Edie's verbal and non-verbal behaviours. For example, if Edie made a vocalisation, ME might attempt to imitate it directly or she might reproduce the rhythm of it in some way, for example by tapping it out on the side of the bed. As such, the investigator would focus on learning Edie's communicative repertoire and reflecting it back to her in a way that was meaningful to Edie.

EDIE'S LANGUAGE

Based on the evidence gathered from the three stages: 1) observation and interviews; 2) baseline interaction and 3) Intensive Interaction, Edie's communication repertoire was found to encompass eye gaze, sound, movements, facial expressions, and several fundamental elements of communication. These are summarized in Table 8.1.

Table 8.1. Edie's communication behaviours

Category	Behaviour		
Eyes	Gaze on partner/partner's eyes	Gaze elsewhere	Eyes closed
Sounds	High-pitched sound	Laughter	Silence
Movements	Sucking and chewing the side of her thumb	Moving her head closer or further away from partner	Moving her head to touch her partner
Facial expressions	Surprise	Smile	Neutral
Fundamental elements	Initiation/introduction of behaviour	Reciprocation of partner's behaviour	Turn taking

We examined the occurrence of these 15 different behaviours across the two one-to-one sessions. The patterns of occurrence of these behaviours were quite different across the two sessions, both in terms of the presence and absence of the behaviours and also in terms of the frequency with which they occurred. To illuminate this difference, the two sessions are briefly described below, starting with the Baseline Interaction. Time checks are included at points where new behaviours occurred or old behaviours ceased in an attempt to clarify the way each session unfolded. In addition, the patterns of occurrence are displayed for each session (see Figure 8.1 and Figure 8.2). For simplicity, these figures are intended as records of whether or not a behaviour occurred during each minute of the two ten-minute sessions; they are not intended to show either counts of frequency nor duration of behaviours.

Session 1: Baseline interaction

When ME entered her room Edie was lying in her bed, which had padded cot-sides. She was lying on her side on two pillows and her eyes were open. When ME asked the first question Edie made a high-pitched sound and stared at her. Edie continued to make the high-pitched sound intermittently whilst looking at ME. Edie's behaviour in response to ME speaking, i.e. making a sound and eye-contact, suggested that she wanted to communicate with her.

At 37 seconds into the session Edie became silent and at 39 seconds into the interaction, she closed her eyes. These behaviours could be taken to indicate disengagement by Edie. However, after a few more seconds she opened her eyes and with a surprised expression made the high-pitched sound. ME continued to ask the prepared questions at 20–second intervals. Edie kept her gaze fixed on ME and at 51 seconds, Edie began chewing her thumb. This activity was one previously identified by Edie's daughter and could serve as a comfort behaviour for Edie (see Chapter 7).

At 62 seconds into the ten-minute session Edie closed her eyes and continued to chew her thumb for another five seconds. She then removed her thumb from her mouth and her eyes remained closed for the rest of the session. ME continued to ask the prepared questions allowing time between each for Edie to respond but *she never again opened her eyes, moved or made a sound* during the remainder of the session.

The total interaction lasted for barely one minute of a planned ten-minute session. The exchange revealed that although Edie appeared to respond to speech at the outset of the session (Figure 8.1), speech alone from her interaction partner failed to maintain her participation. This session confirmed the reports from staff of the difficulties they experienced

Category	Minute	1	2	3	4	5	6	7	8	9
Eyes	Eye-contact with partner	▨								
	Gaze elsewhere									
	Eyes closed		▨	▨	▨	▨	▨	▨	▨	▨
Sound	High-pitched sound	▨								
	Laughter									
	Silence				▨	▨	▨	▨	▨	▨
Movements	Chewing thumb	▨	▨	▨						
	Moving closer/away									
	Touching partner									
Facial expressions	Surprise	▨								
	Smile									
	Neutral				▨	▨	▨	▨	▨	▨
Communication fundamentals	Initiation	▨								
	Reciprocation	▨								
	Turn taking	▨								

Figure 8.1: Presence and absence of Edie's communication behaviours during each minute of the Baseline Session. Shading indicates the behaviour occurred at least once during this minute of the session.

in communicating with Edie in regard to basic activities of daily living. However, the session also contained a number of behaviours, e.g. high-pitched sound and thumb chewing, that Edie's daughter had suggested have a communicative value. These stood out as exactly the sort of behaviours that are used in II to develop an interaction.

Session 2: Intensive Interaction

At the start of this session Edie was lying in her bed with the padded cot-sides. She was lying on her side on two pillows dozing. ME sat by the side of the bed and stroked Edie's hair whilst softly speaking her name. After 16 seconds Edie opened her eyes and looked directly at ME and made 'her' sound in a high-pitched tone. ME reflected the sound and pitch back to Edie. Edie then repeated the sound and both partners took another two turns each in this manner.

As in the Baseline Session, Edie's immediate reaction to ME speaking was to look at her and make the high-pitched sound. In this session, however, rather than continuing to speak, ME adapted her response to match Edie's, which resulted in a brief initial 'dialogue' of several turns each.

At 23 seconds into the interaction, the dialogue changed when Edie put her thumb in her mouth and started sucking and chewing on it, all the time looking into ME's eyes. ME responded by sucking and chewing her thumb. Edie then removed her thumb from her mouth and made her high-pitched sound. ME responded by taking her thumb from her mouth and repeating the sound made by Edie. Edie then put her thumb back into her mouth, and ME followed suit. In these exchanges Edie took the lead by introducing a new behaviour (thumb-chewing), then reverting to the previous behaviour (high-pitched sound) then returning to thumb-chewing, all the time looking intently at ME. ME responded to each of these changes by matching Edie's behaviour.

ME then attempted to change the dialogue by removing her thumb from her mouth and making a sound like Edie's high-pitched one. In response Edie then removed her thumb from her mouth and matched the sound and they then continued to turn take, making this sound for another 20 seconds. This section of dialogue ended when Edie then began sucking her thumb again. In this exchange ME reintroduced one of Edie's behaviours (high-pitched sound) and Edie responded by altering her own behaviour to match ME's.

At 90 seconds into the ten-minute session, ME attempted to change the interaction again by introducing a new element. This was to imitate the rhythm of Edie's thumb chewing through tapping her fingers on the side of the bed. Edie continued to chew her thumb and stared intently at ME. After a few seconds, Edie removed her thumb from her mouth and made her high-pitched sound. ME stopped tapping and repeated the vocal sound and turn-taking resumed using Edie's sound until ME tapped on the bed again. Edie became silent, put her thumb back in her mouth and watched ME's fingers tapping on the bed. She then removed her thumb from her mouth and resumed her high-pitched sound. At 108 seconds, Edie put her thumb in her mouth and immediately removed it when she saw ME do the same. Edie and ME then resumed turn taking with her sound.

In this phase, when ME introduced the new element (rhythmic tapping) there was no discernable change in Edie's behaviour. She continued to chew her thumb while looking intently at ME. However, as ME continued to tap, Edie then stopped chewing and made her high-pitched sound. She did not put her thumb in her mouth again during this session. The turns in this exchange suggest that the introduction of a variation of one her behaviours (thumb-chewing) had less impact for Edie than the matched behaviour. However, she appeared to retain her interest in the interaction as she continued to look at ME and finally reintroduced a previous behaviour (high-pitched sound).

Edie and ME continued the dialogue making the high-pitched sound until 150 seconds into the session, at which point Edie introduced another new behaviour. She lifted her head up from the pillows and moved towards ME's hand, which was resting on the cot-side. Edie rubbed her forehead on ME's hand and ME responded by stroking Edie's hair. ME then attempted to reintroduce one of Edie's previous behaviours, i.e. her thumb-sucking and the rhythm of it. Again, Edie raised her head, rubbed her forehead against ME's hand and then closed her eyes. ME then made Edie's sound towards her to which she reciprocated followed by a number of turns each. Edie continued to keep her eyes closed for 43 seconds during this part of the interaction.

This phase of the session was notable for Edie introducing touch into the interaction. The dialogue had been proceeding through sound and vision (eye-contact) when Edie opened up a third channel of communication, i.e. touch. However, although ME responded by touching Edie's head, she did not match her behaviour, as she had done with Edie's sound.

Category	Minute	1	2	3	4	5	6	7	8	9
Eyes	Eye-contact with partner									
	Gaze elsewhere									
	Eyes closed									
Sound	High-pitched sound									
	Laughter									
	Silence									
Movements	Chewing thumb									
	Moving closer/away									
	Touching partner									
Facial expressions	Surprise									
	Smile									
	Neutral									
Communication fundamentals	Initiation									
	Reciprocation									
	Turn taking									

Figure 8.2: Presence and absence of Edie's communication behaviours during each minute of the Intensive Interaction Session. Shading indicates the behaviour occurred at least once during this minute of the session.

After the sound turn taking, Edie then rubbed her head against ME's hand for a third time and ME moved forward and rubbed her own head against Edie's. At this point, Edie opened her eyes and gave a look of surprise followed by the high-pitched sound. The dialogue then took on the form of a spontaneous game of mutual head touching and vocalisation. During this phase Edie laughed at several points after she and ME touched heads.

This is perhaps the most exciting part of the interaction, as this is when Edie exerted the most control over the situation and was the most animated. Edie was clearly attempting to get closer to ME and to touch her. However, initially ME was focused on maintaining previous elements of the interaction. Once ME recognised Edie's new direction, the interaction took on a new dynamic. From the moment ME touched heads with Edie, communication became much more playful and fun. The two took turns with sounds and touching and both laughed at several points throughout (Figure 8.2).

At seven minutes and four seconds into the interaction, Edie fell silent and closed her eyes. She remained like this until the investigator touched her head 46 seconds later, at which point she made her sound and then opened her eyes when ME reciprocated with the sound. The two began turn taking again using Edie's sound and both laughed several times. At nine minutes and one second, Edie fell silent and then closed her eyes five seconds later. She remained like this for the rest of the session.

This section suggests that perhaps Edie was ready to end the interaction at a point before ME realised. ME attempted to keep the interaction going and Edie reciprocated with enthusiasm for a while but closed her eyes again very soon after. Edie closing her eyes effectively ended the interaction and can be seen as another element of her communication repertoire.

Discussion

This case study reports an attempt to 'learn the language' of Edie, a lady with advanced dementia, using the principles of Intensive Interaction. This approach revealed that Edie retained a varied set of communication behaviours, including eye gaze, movements and sound, coupled with a desire to interact with other people.

At the start of both sessions Edie made eye-contact with the investigator (ME) and a high-pitched sound. In the Baseline 'conversation' Session, however, Edie quickly stopped making any sound or eye-contact and at 67 seconds into the ten minutes, effectively disengaged from the interaction. By contrast, in the II Session the investigator's reciprocation of Edie's initial communication bids led to turn taking and an intricate interaction.

The occurrence of eye-contact and the high-pitched sound at the start of both sessions suggests that in both instances Edie wished to communicate with ME. This confirms earlier findings that the urge to communicate is retained even in the advanced stages of dementia (Astell and Ellis 2006). In addition, when Edie's daughter viewed the videos she reported that this was also how her mother behaved when she visited.

As well as using sound and eye-contact to establish communication, Edie effectively used several different channels of communication during the two interactions with ME. In the Baseline Session she closed her eyes and became silent – i.e. she ceased making her two 'I want to interact' behaviours – very quickly and withdrew from the interaction. By contrast, in the II Session, Edie's high-pitched sound formed the initial exchange with ME, effectively enabling them to say 'hello'.

Throughout the rest of the II Session, Edie used her eyes and her sound to communicate with ME. ME also used the high-pitched sound both in turn taking initiated by Edie and to restore their exchange at several points, e.g. when rhythmic tapping did not elicit a response from Edie. In addition to her eyes and sound, Edie introduced movement and touch, which served to change and intensify the interaction. Once ME reciprocated Edie's touch, the exchange became playful and elicited expression of positive emotion, i.e. laughing.

In addition to new behaviours appearing as the II exchange progressed, it was notable that Edie discontinued chewing her thumb, a behaviour that appeared early in both sessions. Thumb-chewing could serve a number of different functions for Edie. Her daughter, for instance, suggested that it is an indicator of boredom. This fits with the notion that such behaviour is a way that people 'talk to themselves' which enables them to return to their 'comfort zones' (see Chapter 7). It is possible that Edie ceased chewing her thumb during the II Session because she no longer needed to 'talk to herself'. However, in the Baseline Session Edie closed her eyes and became silent when she stopped chewing her thumb. Together these behaviours signalled disengagement and served to terminate her involvement in the interaction. The idea that Edie's behaviour has multiple meanings and that behaviour combining occurs suggests that she retains at least some of the basic components of communication and interaction with another person.

We can see other fundamental aspects of communication behaviour such as initiation, turn taking, using emotional facial expressions (e.g. surprise) and expressing emotion (e.g. laughter) in Edie's communication repertoire. This supports previous findings that even in the advanced stages of dementia, people retain the pre-speech fundamentals of communication (Ellis and Astell 2004; Orange and Purves 1996). In addition, Edie is able to lead the interaction in several different ways. One is by initiating new behaviours, e.g. thumb-sucking, moving towards partner. She is also able to reintroduce old behaviours (thumb-sucking, high-pitched noise) at various points in the interaction. Finally, she is able to end the interaction by closing her eyes and falling silent.

Caregiver reactions

These findings suggest that Edie not only has a retained communication repertoire but also can engage in social interaction and express herself. This was supported by the reaction of Edie's daughter on viewing the video recordings of the two sessions. She confirmed that Edie is very responsive to her when she visits and that her interactions with her mother contain similar elements such as moving her face very close to Edie's. She also reported that holding Edie's hand, cuddling her and talking to her all resulted in what she interpreted to be a happy and animated response. On watching the video recordings, Edie's daughter realised that she copied some of her mother's communicative behaviours when they were interacting without knowing that she was doing it.

Edie's daughter consented to the care home manager viewing the video recordings. The manager's reaction was primarily one of surprise and extreme emotion. She commented that she had never seen Edie communicate so readily and with such obvious engagement. These reactions from Edie's daughter and the care home manager suggest that using the principles of II to facilitate communication between people with advanced dementia such as Edie and those who care for them would indeed be beneficial. In particular, II has the potential for training and supporting care staff, who may find it very difficult to know how to respond to people such as Edie, who make sounds and repetitive behaviours. It could, we hope, give them the confidence to interact with these people who they currently avoid or ignore due to their own discomfort (Kitwood 1990).

Adaptive Interaction

In order to respond to the communication needs of people with advanced dementia some modification of II is required. Specifically, due to the severe memory problems experienced by people with dementia, II with this population must remain 'in the moment' with no need for any parts of previous interactions to be remembered. Therefore, the communication partner must remain adaptive to the changes in communication by the person with dementia and be willing to start afresh each time. As such, we term this approach Adaptive Interaction.

Adaptive Interaction, based on Caldwell's behavioural-matching version of II, appears to have potential as a tool for promoting and supporting communication between people with advanced dementia and those who care for them. This case study uncovered a retained communication repertoire including sounds, movement and eye gaze as well as other basics of communication such as turn taking and facial expressions (Hewett 1996; Nind 1996). Excited by these findings, we are currently exploring the potential of Adaptive Interaction further with five more people with advanced dementia who are no longer able to speak, in the hope of going some way towards bringing them back into the social world.

ACKNOWLEDGEMENTS

We are extremely grateful to Edie and her daughter for participating in this study. We also acknowledge the assistance provided by the manager and staff of the care home where Edie lived. Finally, we are grateful to Phoebe Caldwell for the training and very helpful advice she provided in preparation for carrying out this pilot study. This work was conducted as partial fulfilment of the first author's PhD studies.

Edie recently died very peacefully at the care home she resided in. At her mother's funeral service, Edie's daughter remarked to the minister that although Edie had lost her memory and the ability to speak, dementia could not take away her core humanity. We believe that this chapter illustrates this beautifully and as such dedicate it to Edie's memory and her status as a trailblazer in dementia research.

References

Abad, V. (2002) 'Reaching the socially isolated person with Alzheimer's Disease through group music therapy – A case report.' *Voices: A World Forum for Music Therapy 2*, 3. (GAMUT, Bergen). Accessed on 9/11/07 at www.voices.no/mainissues/Voices2(3)abad.html.

Astell, A.J. and Ellis, M.P. (2006) 'The social function of imitation in severe dementia.' *Infant and Child Development 15*, 311–319.

Bowie, P. and Mountain, G. (1993) 'Using direct observation to record the behaviour of long stay patients with dementia.' *International Journal of Geriatric Psychiatry 8*, 857–864.

Caldwell, P. (2005) *Finding You Finding Me: Using Intensive Interaction to Get in Touch with People whose Severe Learning Disabilities are Combined with Autistic Spectrum Disorder.* Jessica Kingsley Publishers.

Caldwell, P. and Horwood, J. (2007) *From Isolation to Intimacy: Making Friends without Words.* Jessica Kingsley Publishers.

DfES (2001a) *Inclusive Schooling - Children with Special Educational Needs* (ref: DfES/0774/2001). London: DfES.

DfES (2001b) *SEN Toolkit* (ref: DfES 558/2001). London: DfES.

Duffy, M. (1999) 'Reaching the person behind the dementia: Treating co-morbid affective disorders through subvocal and non-verbal strategies.' In M. Duffy (ed.) *Handbook of Counseling and Psychotherapy with Older Adults.* New York: Wiley.

Ellis, M.P. and Astell, A.J. (2004) 'The urge to communicate in severe dementia.' *Brain and Language 91*, 1, 51–52.

Hewett, D. (1996) 'How to do Intensive Interaction.' In M. Collis and P. Lacey (eds) *Interactive Approaches to Teaching: A Framework for INSET.* London: David Fulton Publishers.

Hewett, D. and Nind, M. (eds) (1998) *Interaction in Action: Reflections on the Use of Intensive Interaction.* London: David Fulton Publishers.

Kellett, M. (2000) 'Sam's story: Evaluating intensive interaction in terms of its effect on the social and communicative ability of a young child with severe learning difficulties.' *Support for Learning 15*, 4, 165–171.

Kellett, M. (2003) 'Jacob's journey: Developing sociability and communication in a young boy with severe and complex learning difficulties using the intensive interaction teaching approach.' *Journal of Research in Special Educational Needs 3*, 1, 116–121.

Kitwood, T. (1990) 'The dialectics of dementia: With particular reference to Alzheimer's disease.' *Ageing and Society 10*, 177–196.

Nind, M. (1996) 'Efficacy of Intensive Interaction: Developing sociability and communication in people with severe and complex learning difficulties using an approach based on caregiver–infant interaction.' *European Journal of Special Educational Needs 11*, 1, 48–66.

Nind M. (1999) 'Intensive Interaction and autism: a useful approach?' *British Journal of Special Education 26*, 2, 96–102.

Ofsted (1996/1997) *The Annual Report of Her Majesty's Chief Inspector for Schools: Standards and Quality in Education 1996/97.* London: Stationery Office.

Ofsted (2000) *Writing about Educational Inclusion: Guidance for Inspectors for Writing about Educational Inclusion in Inspection Reports.* www.ofsted.gov.uk/assets/2789.pdf

Orange, J. and Purves, B. (1996) 'Conversational discourse and cognitive impairment: Implications for Alzheimer's disease.' *Journal of Speech-Language Pathology and Audiology 20,* 139–150.

Raia, P. (1999) 'Habilitation Therapy: A New Starscape.' In L. Volicer and L. Bloom-Charette (eds) *Enhancing the Quality of Life in Advanced Dementia.* Philadelphia, PA: Brunner/Mazel.

Samuel, J. and Maggs, J. (1998) 'Introducing Intensive Interaction for People with Profound Learning Disabilities Living in Small Staffed Houses in the Community.' In D. Hewett and M. Nind (eds) *Interaction in Action: Reflections on the Use of Intensive Interaction.* London: David Fulton Publishers.

Stothard, V. (1998) 'The Gradual Development of Intensive Interaction in a School Setting.' In D. Hewett and M. Nind (eds) *Interaction in Action: Reflections on the Use of Intensive Interaction.* London: David Fulton Publishers.

Watson, J. and Fisher, A. (1997) 'Evaluating the effectiveness of Intensive Interaction teaching with pupils with profound and complex learning difficulties.' *British Journal of Special Education 24,* 80–87.

Woods, R.T. (1999) *Psychological problems of ageing: Assessment, treatment and care.* Chichester: Wiley.

PART 3

A Closer Look at Interventions

CHAPTER 9

VIDEO INTERACTION GUIDANCE: A BRIDGE TO BETTER INTERACTIONS FOR INDIVIDUALS WITH COMMUNICATION IMPAIRMENTS

Hilary Kennedy and Heather Sked

This chapter describes the intervention of Video Interaction Guidance (VIG). This is an intervention that seeks to enhance communication and interaction between individuals. It has traditionally been used in a family setting, but is increasingly being used to assist the communication of professionals and clients. Recent innovations with the technique have also begun to explore its application for working with individuals with communicative disorders.

Both authors are educational psychologists. Hilary Kennedy has taught in the Tayside region of Scotland for 24 years, specialising in the assessment of young children with communication and behavioural difficulties. For a considerable portion of this time, she has also led the national training programme for VIG in the UK, which trains professionals in delivering VIG. The second author, Heather Sked, recently completed her MSc in Educational Psychology, and undertook training in VIG while enrolled on that degree.

The chapter is structured in three sections. We begin with a description of VIG, providing a sense of its methods, principles and theoretical base. We then review the growing evidence base that demonstrates VIG's effectiveness for promoting engagement within families and within professional relationships. Finally, we report on a new direction for VIG: its use in the classrooms of children with autism, summarising the findings of a study recently conducted by the second author. This study has particular relevance for this volume because VIG was combined with the technique of imitative responsiveness. This new direction helps to provide a wider vision of the settings in which VIG can be helpful.

Video Interaction Guidance

WHAT IS VIG?

VIG is an intervention that aims to enhance communication within relationships. It is most typically used for interactions between children and adults, either parents or professionals, although it can also be used within pairs (or even groups) of adults. Its aim is to give individuals a chance to reflect on their interactions, drawing attention to elements that are successful and supporting clients to make changes where desired.

Clients are given the opportunity to actively reflect and receive feedback on their interactions by reviewing a microanalysis of video clips of their own successful communication. Before the first session of filming, the client is engaged in the process of change by negotiating his or her own goals. A short (ten minute) film is then taken of the interactions. VIG staff then review this film, with the explicit aim of finding moments within the interaction when the communication between the adult and child is 'more attuned than usual'. Later, the client and facilitator, known in the VIG programme as a 'guide', look together at micro-moments of success. Particular emphasis is placed on moments when the adult has responded in a positive way to the child's action or initiative, using a combination of non-verbal and verbal responses. The client and guide reflect collaboratively on what the pair are doing that is contributing towards the achievement of their goals, they celebrate success and then make further goals for change. These reflections move very quickly from analysis of the behaviour to the exploration of feelings, thoughts, wishes and intentions within the interaction.

The VIG approach takes the view that change can be achieved more effectively in the context of a 'coaching' relationship than 'teaching' relationship, because this is collaborative rather than prescriptive, empowering rather than deskilling. It conveys respect for strengths and potential, rather than drawing attention to problems or weaknesses. Throughout filming and feedback sessions clients are supported to become more sensitive to children's communicative attempts and to develop greater awareness of how they can respond in an attuned way. In the process of standing back and looking at themselves on screen, clients are able to analyse what they were doing when things were going 'better than usual'. In this way they are empowered to make an informed decision about how they would like to improve situations that are more problematic.

The method is based on a model developed in the Netherlands by Harrie Biemans and colleagues over the last 20 years. The concept uses principles which promote successful interactions between mothers and infants in the earliest months as a framework for identifying positive moments in communicative exchanges. These moments are selected by focusing on the way in which children's communicative initiatives are responded to by adults. These principles are fundamental to VIG and are known as the 'contact principles'.

Contact principles relate to the basic building blocks of communication. Although it was developmental psychology, with its emphasis on adult–child relations, that gave birth to these building blocks, through the research paradigms that identified them, the principles can be equally valid in adult client–professional interaction or indeed professional–professional interaction. The building blocks of any communicative interaction are the same: an initiative, a response to that initiative, and an initiative following from that response. Together, these three components equate with taking turns within the communicative process. The development of critical awareness of one's own contribution to this process is a powerful agent towards improved communication ability.

However, the answer to more effective communication does not just lie with an awareness of our own position. A key feature of the communication process is the level of attunement between the communicating parties. We not only have to take account of our own unique style but also that of the person we are communicating with. Trevarthen (1998) refers to such attuned communication as being similar to instruments playing in an orchestra. As he points out in Chapter 2, there is musicality inherent within every successful communication, as those participating must 'play to the beat' while allowing sufficient latitude for creativity and individual style.

THEORETICAL BACKGROUND OF VIG

VIG's 'coaching' focus is on the interaction between people, rather than the behaviour of individuals. The importance of each partner's reception of the other's initiatives, and the natural interaction that develops through turn taking, is the focus for video reflection.

The theoretical underpinning of VIG is based on the work of ethological psychologists such as Daniel Stern (1985) and Colwyn Trevarthen (1979, 1998). Trevarthen drew attention to the types of 'intersubjectivity' that become possible between parents and infants, as infants mature. 'Primary intersubjectivity' is the label now used to describe the process of communication that takes place during the very earliest months, in which emotions are actively expressed and perceived in a two-way dialogue. Very young infants are sensitive to the rhythmic turn taking that sets up the companionship on which the child's social development takes place. Murray and Trevarthen's (1985) work highlighted that as early as two or three months of age, infants are initiating and jointly regulating communicative interactions with other people. Even at this early age, infants are sensitive to, and affected by, the slightest disruption to a two-way dialogue (Nadel *et al.* 1999).

'Secondary intersubjectivity' is characterised by more complex forms of interaction, which become possible during the second half of the first year. By now, infants are able to share a focus with an adult (Hubley and Trevarthen 1979). Objects can now form a focus *between* people, rather than being a focus only for individual members of the dyad. As Hobson (2002) points out, this development implies that an infant is beginning to develop an understanding of the relationship between people and objects. The importance of developing a new shared understanding is a core principle of VIG.

'Mediated learning' also features within the theoretical base of VIG. This term captures the process of a skilled adult guiding a child's activities, but being sure to start from the child's own interests, ability levels and activities. Vygotsky's (1962) concept of the 'Zone of Proximal Development' is relevant here, as he emphasised that the level of support from the adult should be carefully chosen to extend the child from his or her current level but not so advanced that it fails to connect with the child. This process has also been described as 'scaffolding' (Wood, Bruner and Ross 1976), in the context of mother–child interactions.

These ideas are gaining increasing application within the educational setting. Indeed, Jerome Bruner identified them as central to the future direction of the field, in his book *The Culture of Education*: 'The "next" chapter in psychology…is about "intersubjectivity" – how people come to know what others have in mind and how they adjust accordingly' (1996, p.161). Education has only recently refocused on this literature, around the quality of teacher interaction. Alexander's (2004) book *Towards Dialogic Teaching: Rethinking Classroom Talk*, based on rich data from video tapes of classroom interaction in five countries, brings interaction back to the forefront. He develops the Vygotskian view that children construct knowledge from their interaction with more skilled others, thereby putting the relationship between the teacher and the class at the forefront of the educational process. Encouragingly, appreciation of the importance of emotional–expressive dialogue in child development and learning in schools has been given attention in wider contexts, such as the British Psychological Society's declaration of 2005 as the 'Year of the Relationship'.

These, then, are some of the theories that have been most influential in defining the core contact principles used in VIG. These core contact principles provide a framework by which clients, with the assistance of VIG guides, can evaluate their own communication skills during feedback sessions. Examples of the specific application of these principles are shown in Table 9.1.

The evidence base for VIG's effectiveness

The evidence base for the effectiveness of VIG studies has been building up over the last 20 years, through relatively small-scale studies in the Netherlands and the UK. These studies have not only focused on VIG's use with families, its traditional application, but also on its effectiveness for professionals. Both sets of literature will be reviewed here.

VIG AS AN INTERVENTION FOR CHANGE WITH FAMILIES

The first evaluation of VIG in the UK was carried out by Simpson, Forsyth and Kennedy (1995), who measured change in the interaction of five families. The quantitative data obtained from videotapes was triangulated (i.e. compared with) qualitative data obtained by interviewing the families. The study compared the first and final films taken during the VIG programme, and results showed that all the parents became more attuned to their children's initiatives during this period. Their strategies for managing children became more flexible and, although the parents still experienced difficulties, they felt better about how they dealt with them.

It was the positive results of this study that generated the funding for creating the wider VIG project within the UK. There are now over 700

Table 9.1 Contact principles of VIG

Yes-series ATTUNED	Positive responses to child's initiatives	Negative responses to child's initiatives	No-series DISCORDANT
Being attentive	Turn in response Return eye contact	Turning away Looking away	Not attentive
'Yes' giving (body)	Respond with: • smile • nod • friendly intonation • friendly posture	Not smiling Unfriendly intonation Shaking the head Unpleasant facial expression	'No' giving (body)
'Yes' giving (verbal)	Talking Labelling Saying yes Each making initiatives Saying what you feel Asking what you want to know	Remaining silent Correcting Saying no	'No' giving (verbal)
Taking turns	Receiving and returning	Everyone talking at once Not receiving Not taking a turn	Not taking turns

Cooperation		Not cooperating	
	Receiving		Not receiving help
	Giving help		Not giving help
			Not joining in
Attuned guiding, leading	Taking initiatives	Discordant guiding, leading	Not taking initiatives
	Distracting		Not distracting
	Making suggestions		Not making suggestions
	Making choices		Not making choices
	Making plans		Not making plans
	Problem solving		Not problem solving

trained VIG practitioners and 50 supervisors working in almost all governmental regions in Scotland. VIG is also now gaining strength in the southeastern regions of England, with projects emerging in the Midlands and Newcastle.

Two reviews of developments since 1995 have recently been published. The first is by Paul Wels in his book *Helping with a Camera: The Use of Video for Family Intervention* (2002). He highlights the multiple ways in which video systems are now used to support families. The second review is a meta-analysis by Fukkink (2007) of 28 studies (with a total of 1794 families) carried out to assess the effectiveness of VIG in the UK and the Netherlands. This review showed statistically significant effects of this approach on parenting behaviour: 'Parents became more skilled at interacting with their young child and experience fewer problems in and gain more pleasure in their role as a parent and attitude of parents and the development of the child' (Fukkink 2007, Abstract). Interestingly, the effect was greater when the intervention was shorter and was focused on specific behavioural elements. Not surprisingly, the results for children of parents in high-risk groups were less favourable than those in lower-risk groups.

Fukkink (2007) went on to conduct a supplementary analysis, in which he compared the effect size of VIG with other family support programmes. This is summarised in Table 9.2. The results show a trend toward a superior effect size, although it did not achieve statistical significance.

Table 9.2 Effect sizes of VIG compared with other programmes

Effect size	Parental behaviour	Parental attitude	Child's behaviour
VIG	0.76	0.56	0.42
Other programmes	0.47	0.24	0.29

Source: Fukkink 2007

Overall, these data sets indicate that VIG has considerable potential as an intervention for change, and that closer analysis would benefit our understanding of how the programme functions differently in the Netherlands and the UK, so that we can gain a better understanding of how to extend its helpfulness to a greater range of families.

VIG AS A TOOL FOR TRAINING PROFESSIONALS

In the last five years VIG has been adapted for use as a staff training method in educational, medical and social work settings. In 2001 Dundee Educational Psychology Service and Pre-school Home Visiting Service presented a training course called 'Addressing the emotional and communication needs of young children: How to use the contact principles and keep in the yes-cycle!' The course involves each participant making three videos of themselves communicating with young children, and then creating their own plan for change. Over half of the 270 professionals to whom presentations about this course have been made have now taken up the offer of VIG coaching sessions. Those who have completed it have consistently accorded it positive evaluations (Kennedy 2005).

Fukkink and Tavecchio (2007) carried out an assessment of this professional invention, evaluating interactions filmed in day-care settings. The evaluation was conducted blind, with the researchers unaware of whether the sessions being assessed represented pre- or post-intervention periods. Results showed an increase in sensitivity, responsivity and language stimulation in caregivers' interaction with the children, following training. These improvements were still visible three months after intervention.

The above evaluations give a strong mandate for the effectiveness of the delivery of three to four coaching sessions in VIG, as a means of promoting measurable, positive change in professionals' interactions with children.

Using VIG to improve interactions with children with Autism Spectrum Disorder

A recent development of the use of VIG was undertaken by Heather Sked (second author of this chapter) in supporting the communicative interactions of children with autism and their educational staff (Sked 2006). Children with Autistic Spectrum Disorder (ASD) are described as lacking intersubjective contact (Hobson 2002). This may help to explain why children with ASD have difficulty developing language, for social and emotional engagement provide the basis for linguistic development. Enhancing such engagement is exactly what VIG aims to achieve. This makes VIG well suited to the problems faced by children with ASD. In this study, we combined VIG with an intervention of imitative responsiveness, similar to that described by Jacqueline Nadel (Nadel and Pezé 1993), whose data clearly show that children with ASD who have previously been unavailable for interaction become much more socially engaged, following imitation sessions with an adult. (A similar set up is described in Chapter 4.) We believed that combining VIG with this imitation technique was likely to heighten the positive outcomes that have been previously reported by such authors.

Case studies of six boys of primary school age on the autistic spectrum were undertaken. Each child and his educational auxiliary worker participated in five play sessions. In the first session, the adults interacted with the children as normal, and in the later sessions, the adults were encouraged to respond to the children using imitation. To facilitate imitation, dual sets of toys were provided during play sessions, following the procedures established by Nadel and Pezé (1993) and O'Neill (2007). The sessions were filmed, and in each of the first four sessions the adults also took part in VIG feedback sessions. Discussion in the sessions focused on the balance between the auxiliary's and the child's use of the contact principles.

The effectiveness of this intervention was assessed by tracking changes in the interaction within dyads over the five sessions. The multiple case analysis permitted by this study design was particularly well suited to such an examination, as it presented the opportunity to look for trends both across the group and within dyads. Two research questions were posed. First, did interaction improve when the adult imitated the child's actions in a play situation? Second, did interaction improve further when the adult received VIG feedback on the interaction? These questions were addressed by coding one minute's worth of interaction from each of the five sessions. The incidence of four specific aspects of communication that relate to the VIG contact principles were coded on a second-by-second basis. These were: direction of gaze, focus of action, verbal contributions, and expressions of pleasure. Sessions typically lasted 10 minutes or longer. For the purpose of analysis, we chose to examine behaviours that occurred during the 60-second period between 4.01 and 5.00 minutes, given that this period fell in the middle of the session.

Several other methods of analysis were employed for triangulation purposes. A disinterested third party rated the 'attunement' of each dyad, in a randomly ordered presentation of films for sessions 1 (no imitation), 2 and 5. The staff were also asked to complete questionnaires at the beginning and end of the study which allowed us to gain insights into their experience of and attitudes toward this intervention. Finally, the discussions that took place during VIG feedback sessions were recorded (on video), and the contents of the discussion were then analysed to identify the extent to which staff made any spontaneous mention of changes that they observed in the children's behaviour which they attributed to the use of imitation. We hoped that they might spontaneously identify the kinds of changes described by Caldwell (2006) in her use of Intensive Interaction, including greater attention to the adult partner, calmer behaviour and more positive emotion.

A full account of the findings of this complex study can be obtained from Sked (2006). A flavour of the outcomes will be presented here.

Figures 9.1 and 9.2 show behavioural outcomes for four of the children. These four children provide an interesting contrast between those who demonstrated reasonable linguistic ability (N=3) and those who had less (N=1). The results for the three children with linguistic ability are shown in Figure 9.1 (Children A, B and C). They show that, in all cases, the adult decreased his or her verbal contributions following training in imitation (Film 2 versus Film 1). They also show that the children gradually made more verbal contributions (Films 3, 4 and 5), and that as the child's verbal contributions increased the adult's contributions also began to gradually increase.

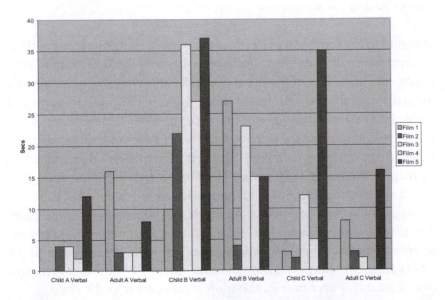

Figure 9.1: Changes in verbal contributions of adults and children over the five intervention sessions, for children with greater linguistic capacity (N=3)

Results for the child who showed least linguistic ability (Child D) are shown in Figure 9.2. Because of this low linguistic ability, his progress is illustrated with the variable direction of gaze. A marked increase can be seen in both his and the adult worker's gaze to a toy that was the object of joint gaze.

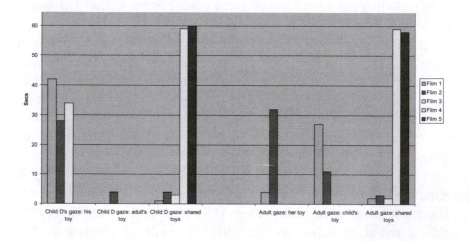

Figure 9.2: Changes in direction of gaze for adult and child over the five intervention sessions, for the child with least linguistic capacity (N=1)

In regard to the third-party ratings of attunement, judgements were that a clear increase in the adult's attunement to the child could be seen for three dyads, over the course of the five sessions. Results were more conflicted in the remaining three dyads. Importantly, though, there were no dyads in which adult attunement was not found to increase at some point. When the pattern of attunement development was investigated in more detail, two patterns could be identified. The first pattern showed an immediate increase in attunement, following Session 2 when imitation was introduced, with further increases in attunement in the sessions that followed. This pattern applied to three of the dyads. In the remaining three dyads, the increase in attunement was less sharp, demonstrating a more gradual improvement over the five sessions. In no case, however, did improvements cease after the first session of imitation; in all cases there were continued increases over time in the adult's attunement to the child.

It is possible that increased experience of imitation sessions stimulated development of attunement. This interpretation would accord with other studies that have demonstrated increases in social interaction for children with ASD over repeated imitation sessions (e.g. Nadel and Pezé 1993; O'Neill 2007). It is also possible that, through VIG feedback, increased awareness of the child's needs stimulated the staff member's development of attunement, which in turn produced more attuned behaviour on the part of children. Alternatively, increased awareness of the child's developing attunement may have stimulated changes in the staff member's behaviour.

It is also interesting to consider these VIG feedback sessions from the social constructionist perspective espoused by Simpson *et al.* (1995). From a social constructionist perspective, the self is multi-faceted. The relationship between the researcher and each of the auxiliaries was emergent and contextual. That is, the understanding between the researcher and each auxiliary of the effect of imitation was mutually developed in each case, emerging from contextual discussion with relation to the specific child. In addition, each auxiliary's experience of using imitation occurred within a contextual relationship with the child. The experience of each case study was genuinely exploratory and inevitably unique. Attitudes to smaller behavioural changes seemed to be influenced by the relationships and by the way that the staff attributed their success or otherwise.

All auxiliaries stated (in either feedback or questionnaires) that they would consider using imitation as a communicative strategy in future. They could all identify situations when they felt it might be useful. This was notable because facilitating ongoing change in practice had not been an aim of this study. A significant factor here may be that five of the six auxiliaries spontaneously mentioned behaviour changes which Caldwell (2000) noted as possible outcomes of the use of imitative interventions, including attention to the partner and positive emotions. Three of the auxiliaries also commented on the intervention's usefulness in managing the child's emotions and sensory state, helping 'to calm him down', 'to put him in a better frame of mind', 'when he becomes anxious'. Using imitation with the child had allowed them to experience its effect, and VIG feedback had allowed them to reflect upon that experience and make it explicit. Furthermore, VIG feedback offered the opportunity to explore implications of imitation, including the use of surprise, swapping the lead roles, and exploring the emotional impact of imitation (Caldwell 2006;

Zeedyk 2006). In all these ways the use of imitation had the potential to meet immediate needs in the workplace and VIG feedback offered the opportunity to make this explicit. Where auxiliaries found this to be the case, they seemed particularly inclined towards further exploration of the potential benefits of imitation through the process of filming and feedback.

Final reflections

The effectiveness of VIG is influenced greatly by the quality of the relationship between the client and the VIG guider. This can be seen over the case studies examined in this study. The engagement of the auxiliaries in the process of self-reflection and change during the VIG video feedback sessions was qualitatively different. Some were highly emotionally engaged in the process of change and, not surprisingly, those auxiliaries were the ones who experienced successful new connections with the child in the film. They could see for themselves that following the child's lead helped the child 'feel their presence' and could support the child in making new initiatives. The reviewing of these 'moments of contact' had a profound emotional effect on these staff members. The films of their video feedback sessions demonstrate their increase in confidence, enthusiasm and the new ideas they brought to the interaction, which in turn led to enhanced two-way communication. These shifts were less obvious, and less effective, for auxiliaries who were less emotionally engaged in the process of change.

When looking at the quality of the staff's engagement with and 'imitation' of the child, there was huge variability in the emotional quality of their interactions. Imitation can be a 'wooden' exact copying, or it can be a 'flowing dance', with elements of surprise and fun. Caldwell (2006) would argue that mere copying is inadequate, and indeed insulting, as a form of intervention. What imitative techniques should promote is creative responsiveness – doing with, rather than doing to. Zeedyk's (2006) revised definition of imitation as 'mirroring, mimicking, copying, emulation, co-action and joining, indeed any activity/state in which *the focus of the attention is the partner*' (p.334) highlights these nuances in the definition and practice of imitation.

Lambert (1992) has argued that the quality of relationships and extratherapeutic factors are key to the success of interventions. We believe that is certainly the case with VIG. Lambert's findings showed that the actual model of intervention accounts for only 15 per cent of the change process, with the relationship between therapist and client, as well as activation of client factors, accounting for approximately 70 per cent of the change. It follows then that the quality of the feedback process will be central to the success of VIG as an intervention. The emergent relationship continually developing between the researcher and each auxiliary teacher taking part in this study would shape the experience of the imitation sessions for each auxiliary and child. Conversely, the emergent relationship between the adult and child would influence the quality of the feedback sessions. This may seem like common sense, as we all know that the first few minutes with a doctor determine how much we can get out of a short consultation. However, such interpersonal factors can easily be overlooked in designing and evaluating interventions.

VIG is not a simple skills-based training that can be learnt by following a manual. The training process for professionals provides an in-depth focus on the developing relationship between professional and client. The supervision sessions on the video feedback give space for self-reflection, support in developing plans for improvement and opportunities for recognising change on the video. This cyclical process has all the elements of effective adult learning. Supervisors see their VIG trainees becoming more animated and effective with their clients as they progress through the training. Many VIG practitioners will state that this way of working has fundamentally changed their interactions at work. This helps to explain why there is such a high level of enthusiasm and dedication to this way of working expressed by those involved, and why the feedback from clients who have taken part in VIG sessions remains so consistently positive.

References

Alexander, R. (2004) *Towards Dialogic Teaching: Rethinking Classroom Talk*. Cambridge: Dialogos.

Bruner, J.S. (1996) *The Culture of Education*. Cambridge, MA: Harvard University.

Caldwell, P. (2000) *You Don't Know What it's Like*. Brighton: Pavilion Publishing (Brighton) Ltd.

Caldwell, P. (2006) *Finding You, Finding Me: Using Intensive Interaction to Get in Touch with People whose Severe Learning Disabilities are Combined with Autistic Spectrum Disorder*. London: Jessica Kingsley Publishers.

Fukkink, R.G. (2007) *Video Feedback in the Widescreen: A Meta-analysis of the Effects of Video Feedback in Family Programmes* (SCO report 767, project number 40128). Amsterdam: SCO-Kohnstamm Instituut, University of Amsterdam.

Fukkink, R.G. and Tavecchio, L.W.C. (2007) 'Effects of video interaction analysis in a childcare context'. *Pedagogische Studiën 84*, 1, 55–70.

Hobson, P. (2002) *The Cradle of Thought.* Oxford: Macmillan.

Hubley, P. and Trevarthen, C. (1979) 'Sharing a Task in Infancy.' In I.C. Uzgiris (ed.) *Social Interaction and Communication During Infancy.* San Francisco: Jossey Bass.

Kennedy, H. (2005) 'Film focus: Improving adults communication with children.' *Children in Scotland*, November.

Lambert, M.J. (1992) 'Implications of Outcome Research for Psychotherapy Integration.' In J.C. Norcross and M.R. Goldfried (eds) *Handbook of Psychotherapy Integration.* New York: Basic Books.

Murray, L. and Trevarthen, C. (1985) 'Emotional Regulation of Interactions between Two-month-olds and their Mothers.' In T.M. Field and N.A. Fox (eds) *Social Perspectives in Infants.* Norwood, NJ: Ablex.

Nadel, J., Carchon, I., Kervella, C., Marcelli, D. and Reserbat-Plantey, D. (1999) 'Expectancies for social contingency in 2-month-olds.' *Developmental Science 2*, 2, 164–173.

Nadel, J. and Pezé, A. (1993) 'What Makes Immediate Imitation Communicative in Toddlers and Autistic Children?' In J. Nadel and L. Camaioni (eds) *New Perspectives in Early Communicative Development.* London: Routledge.

O'Neill, M.B. (2007) 'Imitation as an intervention for children with Autistic Spectrum Disorder and their parents/carers.' PhD thesis, University of Dundee.

Simpson, R., Forsyth, P. and Kennedy, H. (1995) *An Evaluation of Video Interaction Analysis in Family and Teaching Situations.* Professional Development Initiatives. SED/Regional Psychological Services.

Sked, H. (2006) 'Learning their language: A comparative study of social interactions between children with autism and adults, using imitation and Video Interaction Guidance as interventions.' Thesis submitted in part fulfilment of an MSc in Educational Psychology, University of Dundee.

Stern, D. (1985) *The Interpersonal World of the Child.* New York: Basic Books.

Trevarthen, C. (1979) 'Communication and Co-operation in Early Infancy: A Description of Primary Intersubjectivity.' In M. Bullowa (ed.) *Before Speech.* Cambridge: Cambridge University Press.

Trevarthen, C. (1998) 'The Concept and Foundations of Infant Intersubjectivity.' In S. Braten (ed.) *Intersubjective Communication and Emotion in Early Ontogeny.* Cambridge: Cambridge University Press.

Vygotsky, L.S. (1962) *Thought and Language.* Cambridge, MA: MIT Press. (Original work published 1934.)

Wels, P. (2002) *Helping with a Camera: The Use of Video for Family Intervention.* Nijmegen: Nijmegen University Press.

Wood, D., Bruner, J.S. and Ross, G. (1976) 'The role of tutoring in problem-solving.' *Journal of Child Psychology and Psychiatry 17*, 89–100.

Zeedyk, M.S. (2006) 'From intersubjectivity to subjectivity: The transformative roles of emotional intimacy and imitation.' *Infant and Child Development 15*, 321–344.

CHAPTER 10

SENSORY INTEGRATION: FROM SPINNING TO SITTING, FROM SITTING TO SMILING

Jane Horwood

All of us have some ability to make sense of and to process the intensity, amount and type of sensation impinging on our bodies. This results in responses and behaviours that can appear either organised or disorganised. This chapter will explore the topics of sensory processing and sensory integration, which offer ways of thinking about the organisation of sensory input. It will look particularly at the relationship of sensory integration to an individual's ability to engage with his or her environment and to be available for communication. Understanding sensory processing and integration helps us to develop interventions that can be used to help individuals when the world appears a disorganised chaos of sensation.

The chapter will summarise the theory of Sensory Integration. This theory draws attention to the sensory stimulation that often goes unnoticed. For example, as well as the senses of sight, smell, taste and hearing, our tactile sense provides information to the brain concerning pain, temperature and vibration, as well as the different forms of touch that are possible. Additional sensory systems – vestibular and proprioceptive – provide information to the brain regarding gravity, muscle tension, joint position and the perception of movement. When we pay more attention to these sensory systems, we often have deeper insights into a person's behaviour – including our own. I will go on to describe how the theory of Sensory Integration can be used to reduce sensory overload, to facilitate the integration of sensory systems and to assist individuals in being available for communication. These shifts allow individuals to engage more readily with the world around them.

I am a paediatric occupational therapist. I work with children of any age (0–19 years) and their families and carers, in educational, home or other relevant settings. Through postgraduate training and facilitation of therapy sessions with individuals, I have learnt how important it is both to understand and appreciate the impact that poor sensory processing and dysfunctional sensory integration can have on our ability to function, learn and develop. When individuals exhibit difficulty in engaging in the world, as those with special needs, learning difficulties and autism often do, then this understanding allows me to develop hypotheses about what their sensory processing is like. From that basis, an intervention plan can be put in place to alleviate any sensory distress they are experiencing.

The origins of Sensory Integration

Dr A. Jean Ayres proposed the theory of Sensory Integration in the 1970s in the United States (Ayres 1979). Originally she directed her theory towards those people with specific learning and behavioural difficulties. But by the late 1980s she had recognised that Sensory Integration and its intervention techniques applied equally to individuals with neuro-developmental disabilities. Other theorists have subsequently applied the principles of Sensory Integration Theory to patients with neuro-motor disorders. Research into Autistic Spectrum Disorders and associated deficits in imitation, interaction and social communication has for some time identified problems with sensory processing which impact upon social interaction and social responses (e.g. Baraneck 1999; Dawson and Adams 1984; Osterling and Dawson 1994). The presence of sensory processing deficits in children (and adults) with cerebral palsy is now also well supported in literature (Cooper et al. 1995; Lesny et al. 1993). Sensory Integration and its intervention techniques thus apply to a wide range of people – indeed to all of us. One need not have 'special needs' to benefit from a better of understanding Sensory Integration, as I will go on to show.

Understanding Sensory Integration

I am a clinician. Sensory Integration Theory and its interventions allow me to look at an individual's behaviour from 'a sensory point of view'. It permits alternative interpretations of self-stimulatory and/or self-abusing behaviours. It lets me ask: why does one individual need to touch everything and everyone to the point of irritation, whereas another, with a matching diagnostic label, withdraws to a corner of the room, avoiding touch in any form? Or: how could an individual possibly follow a verbal instruction or interact with another person when all he or she can attend to is the overwhelming sensation of a label in his or her shirt? Sensory Integration Theory interventions make us, as practitioners, more aware of these sensory issues, and help us to develop means of providing sensory input that can calm individuals and aid their central nervous system organisation.

My practice makes me aware that, for an individual with poor sensory integration, the world can feel a disorganised, distressing place. Sensitivity to light, discomfort with the textures of clothing next to the skin, sensitivity to certain sounds, and similar sensations all add to heightened anxieties, feelings of being overwhelmed and general discomfort within the environment. Here are some examples, drawn from my own experience, that show the real consequences of these sensory experiences:

> Julie, a baby with sensory integration difficulties, is not calmed by being held by her mother. Holding is interpreted by her as 'threatening'. Her protective tactile response system overreacts, and she arches her back to try to ease her discomfort, squirming and crying.

> Sam, a pre-schooler, stops at the edge of the pavement, unable to step off the kerb to cross the road with his mother. He is overwhelmed by the sensation of disorientation that a change in body position causes him every time he steps up and down a kerb or step. He freezes, unable to move.

> Harriet, who is on the autistic spectrum, circles her classroom, visually monitoring all that is going on. She flits from activity to activity, unable to engage for more than a few seconds at a time with anyone or anything. As long as Harriet keeps moving, she can just about cope with the noise of the classroom. When she stands still, the noise is too much. So, trying to block out painful noise sensations, Harriet covers her ears with her hands and screams, making her own noise to blot out the classroom noise.

> Adam, a child of primary school age, is non-verbal, passive and unresponsive. Without prompting from the adults around him, he may stop mid-mouthful when feeding himself, unable to put the spoon in his mouth, despite the fact that it is loaded with a chosen

favourite food. It may be hypothesised that Adam's difficulties
with registering sensory input directly impact upon his ability to
carry out basic motor actions consistently and successfully.

These examples show how, from a Sensory Integration point of view, we
depend on the sensory information we receive from our bodies and the
environment to make sense of the world around us. If such information is
(mis)interpreted by our brains, for whatever reason, as uncomfortable,
painful or confusing, we may then preferentially attend to very specific
sensations to try to provide a stimulus that our brain *can* understand, and
even use this specific sensation to block out the uncomfortable, painful
and confusing sensations around us.

Let me give some more examples.

> James is a non-verbal individual on the autistic spectrum who
> makes frequent clicks and whistles with his mouth and tongue
> when placed in a noisy, busy or new environment. It appears that
> the mouth vibrations caused by clicking and the 'muscle work' of
> whistling give James sensory input that is calming, organising and
> meaningful to him. James is perhaps using his own noise to block
> out noises which are painful to his over-sensitive auditory system,
> thereby providing his own vibratory, proprioceptive input.

> Jimmy is 14 years old. Repeatedly, he engages in hitting people
> and throwing objects. He smiles as he smacks the leg of a passing
> adult, enjoying the vibratory sensation as it moves up his arm. If
> he hits or throws hard enough, his joints will even experience a
> jarring sensation. Jimmy does not like light touch or engaging in
> discriminatory touch experiences. The additional proprioceptive
> input he receives from jarring his joints appears to calm his
> over-responsive tactile system.

Sensory integration can be a complex process to understand, especially if
'the rest of us' tend to experience coherent sensory integration each day
on an unconscious basis. When a fly lands on our arm, our brain is able to
locate where the additional sensory input is coming from. It sorts and
organises that information in order that our body can move, behave and
react appropriately. When the brain does not experience problems in
sensory integration, it can perform such organisation unconsciously. But
when the brain does have trouble sorting such information, then it
becomes stuck in an endless rush-hour traffic jam, as Jean Ayres (1979)

puts it. The constant flow of sensory information begins to be perceived as threatening and/or confusing.

Sensory Integration in practice

When I am putting these insights into practice in my clinical work, I take time to observe individuals in their environment(s). I ask myself to notice, for example:

- What sensory input are they seeking or avoiding?

- Do they appear to be registering specific sensory input?

- When and in what situation do they withdraw or engage in inappropriate behaviours?

- When is the individual happiest, most calm and best organised?

Standardised tests can also be used. Jean Ayres developed the Sensory Integration and Praxis Test (SIPT; Ayres 1989). Winnie Dunn has gone on to develop a standardised questionnaire for carers, entitled the Sensory Profile (Dunn 1999). However, I would suggest that timely observation and discussion with parents, carers and teachers is often as useful as these standardised measures.

Ayres estimated that 5–10 per cent of 'normal children' experience sensory integration problems that would benefit from intervention. Such problems interfere with the child's ability to participate in and perform the 'normal' activities of childhood. Look at your friends and family. The efficiency of sensory processing varies from individual to individual. Some of us have natural athletic ability, easily learn new skills and adapt to change well. Others may take time to learn a new routine in an aerobics class or to learn to drive a car. Others may not cope well with change to their routine or they dislike busy shopping centres. We have all probably put away a jumper into the back of a drawer because it is 'too itchy to wear'.

Perhaps now you prefer to hold the coats when the family visits a fair or leisure park, whereas previously, as an adolescent, you craved the sensation of being whirled round and round. When I feel stressed, sometimes even the sound of a voice asking me a question is enough to cause an emotional response, even though the words in the question are simply

'Would you like a cup of tea?' All of us are individuals with particular sensory needs and varying efficiencies of sensory processing. This is the awareness I bring with me each time I meet a new client – that each person has different thresholds for processing sensory information. We are all 'disabled' in some way or another.

Integration of senses

Donna Williams (1998), an adult on the autistic spectrum, comments that if she cuts down her visual sensory overload by wearing coloured lenses in glasses, she can process auditory information more successfully. By desensitising one sensory input, we appear to allow space for other sensations to process appropriately. This is an important element in understanding sensory integration and how it relates to each of us.

Nothing works in isolation. If I pick up my pet rabbit, my proprioceptive sense allows me to use the correct force and effort so that I do not hurt the animal. My tactile sense enjoys the experience of soft fur, but additionally helps me to know where my fingers are when vision is blocked. Visually, I monitor whether the rabbit is restless. I listen for noises that I interpret as meaning 'put me down'. Meanwhile, my vestibular sense helps me to stand still and balance whilst holding the weight of the rabbit. I am in a calm state, appropriate for handling a small, furry animal.

Conversely, if I passed the rabbit to Jimmy, whom I described above, his poor vestibular processing may make it necessary for him to keep moving whilst holding the rabbit. In order to know where his limbs are in space, Johnny may end up using too much force and squash the poor rabbit, ultimately dropping it abruptly when suddenly touching its ear! He is unable to respond automatically, efficiently and comfortably to the sensory input he received in his 'rabbit encounter'.

I am able to interpret the sensory information from stroking a rabbit and compare such a new sensory experience with old sensory experiences. Language, memory and the brain's emotional centres are all involved with this interpretation process. Touching the rabbit reminded me of a visit to Pets Corner at a local zoo in my childhood – a pleasant experience. My central nervous system, programmed to sensory input which will 'keep me safe', interpreted the stroking of the rabbit as non-threatening. However, Jimmy's over-responsive tactile protection system would not enable him to react in the same pleasant manner. His system would react to the touch sensation of the rabbit's ear with a 'fright, fight, or flight' response. Thus, the meaning that a stimulus holds (i.e., in this case a rabbit's ear) lies not in the stimulus itself, but in the way each of us are able to interpret and respond to that stimulus.

Looking at Jimmy's behaviour with 'sensory glasses' on, we develop a better understanding of his behaviours and his levels of anxiety. We are then able to work with Jimmy to alleviate his sensory difficulties and to support him, respectfully, in being able to have new experiences of the world.

Sensory experiences

If atypical language, memory and development are present in an individual, then a sensory experience may not be adequately stored or remembered. Pleasant sensory experiences may not be connected with positive emotions. If sensory input is inconsistent and/or distorted, sensory interpretation can be hampered. Information may not even register.

When I am stressed (as my family knows too well!), I become controlling and obsessed with the cleanliness of our home. Many individuals with sensory integration dysfunction become stubborn and controlling too, in their efforts to keep the input to the central nervous system predictable. Transitions and changes in their daily schedule become a battleground, a time of increased anxiety, as they become overwhelmed with new sensory sensations they are unable to make sense of. Familiarity – keeping everything the same – is a method of reducing sensation when sensation is repeatedly interpreted as unfamiliar.

If we are on 'sensory alert' then high levels of anxiety reign supreme. When we are stressed or highly anxious, our neurological thresholds for sensory information diminish. Normally, I can cope with two or three people speaking at once. When stressed, however, my neurological threshold for auditory information is lowered and even the kind verbal offer 'Would you like a cup of tea?' can be interpreted by me as threatening or overwhelming. I react verbally and withdraw from the situation.

I have learnt that there are sensory inputs which help me cope when stressed or overwhelmed by other sensory experiences. Engaging in any type of physical activity – a walk, a bike ride or a trip to the gym – can help me to decrease my hyper-reactive responses to sensory input and to feel calmer and more organised. Some children use excessive movement or their own expressive noise to help screen out irritating or uncomfortable sensory input.

When sensory integration is functioning, our brains can respond in a physical, emotional and cognitive manner. For example, I realise that I can choose to ignore the question 'Would you like a cup of tea?' I recognise my emotional response of anxiety, and I respond by physically moving away and making my excuses to the individuals involved.

Non-verbal children in a classroom setting often do not have these options. They have no safe place to retreat to, and thus display fright, fight and flight responses – unsurprising, given that they are unable to demonstrate a cognitive response, unable to enact their own emotional wellbeing, and unable physically to withdraw.

As the sensory situation becomes overwhelming, the child's breathing rate increases. He becomes restless and agitated. He may engage in self-stimulatory behaviours, such as hand biting or head banging. Such behaviours are noticed by the adult in charge and she approaches, thereby invading the child's personal space. Now the child is in full fright, fight and flight mode and, in a last ditch effort to withdraw, hits out.

Atypical emotional development and cognitive development may interfere further with the response open to individuals. The physical or emotional response that they offer may be out of proportion to the situation or, conversely, too minimal to match that introduced by their partner. For example, if someone hits Jimmy, his tactile and proprioceptive systems appear not to register such sensory input. He under-responds. Jimmy doesn't even seem to notice he has been hit. Another child may go into complete meltdown over a simple paper cut!

Impaired sensory processing or sensory integration also impacts on motor planning. Motor planning is the ability to anticipate, initiate and execute a motor response. Offered a box of chocolates, I am able to reach out to pick up my desired chocolate. Some children, though, have difficulty starting, stopping or changing motor actions. They appear non-compliant when given a motor-related instruction, or they resort to self-stimulatory behaviours. Greenspan and Wieder (1997) reported on 200 cases of children on the autistic spectrum. All the children experienced some sort of motor planning problem.

When sensory integration is working well we are able to balance our emotional responses, attend to the task in hand, plan and carry out the motor aspects of the task efficiently, filter out any unnecessary sensory input and control our impulses until the task is completed. We can sit quietly in a church service, then jump up and down cheering loudly at a rugby match. We can run around the garden madly with a new puppy, then quietly sit and listen to a friend in crisis on the phone. Children with sensory processing problems are often not in the right state of arousal for the task or situation they are in and require additional adult intervention.

Let me give some examples of when such intervention would be helpful.

> Harriet is unable to sit still and participate in 'circle time' at school until she undertakes a period of vigorous physical activity. Only then is she in a ready state for the required activity.

> Babies and young children can be observed trying to self-calm, regulating their own levels of arousal through thumb-sucking, stroking a comfort blanket, or twirling their own hair.

> Other children remain in a state of high arousal, unable to self-calm, without the attention of an adult to, perhaps, encourage them to sit down, rub their back to relax their breathing, and talk in a rhythmic fashion to them in order to get them to focus on other sensations.

> My son, as a baby, suffered from frequent ear infections. He was unable to self-calm or even begin to regulate his own levels of arousal. The only way to get him to sleep was to put a hairdryer on for 20–30 minute periods, providing his brain with monotonous, overwhelming noise. When placed in his pram, we shook and rocked the pram violently, supplying our own 'earthquake intervention'. His sister emerged into the world two years later and immediately placed her thumb in her mouth. She had discovered her ability to self-calm in utero, I surmise. As a young child, my son found it difficult to amuse himself. He sought out adult intervention. My daughter would quite happily sit in her high chair with a box of raisins and a good view of the world, quite content.

We are all unique in respect of our sensory motor preferences, our ability to self-regulate, and our capacity to utilise sensory input successfully. Even within the same family, sensory differences can be notable.

With such differences in mind, Williams and Shellenberger (1994) have developed a programme that teaches self-regulation strategies, called 'How Does Your Engine Run?' The programme teaches adults and children to recognise their own levels of 'engine speed' (i.e. alertness) and then implement strategies which assist the matching of the engine speed (that is, the level of alertness) to the task in hand. The development of this programme reminds us that it is not just adults and children with 'disorders' who would benefit from intervention programmes. All of us benefit when we have a better understanding of sensory processes.

Sensory Integration interventions

Sensory Integration Theory does more than increase our understanding of people's behaviour. It also provides specific strategies which help individuals to achieve a state of calmness, alertness, and a readiness to engage with their environment and be available for communication.

Harriet, as previously described, is unable to sit still at early morning circle time in her classroom, because she needs urgently to move around when she arrives at school. But when we introduce Sensory Integration sessions specifically designed for Harriet, where she can, for example, go round and round on a tyre swing for 20 minutes or so, then she is readily able to engage in sedentary educational activities. Left solely to her own devices, Harriet is unable to be in a 'just right' state of arousal on a consistent basis. She cannot filter out and balance incoming sensory information without adult intervention. With the input of Sensory Integration techniques, Harriet is available to re-engage with her environment and the people in it. We have been working with Harriet over a period of time now, using an ongoing programme of Sensory Integration activities, with the very positive outcome being that she is better able to engage with her environment, and her levels of verbal and non-verbal communication continue to improve.

The needs of some children can be met through parents, teachers and carers incorporating specified sensory activities into their daily schedule. Other children require more extensive Sensory Integration Therapy, with an experienced occupational therapist, in order to facilitate more functional responses to sensory stimuli. In my clinical work, I aim to put together programmes, or 'sensory diets', of such strategies, specialised for each child. Parents, carers and school staff are then given training both formally and informally in order to be able to fully integrate such strategies in the child's everyday life.

The aim of this approach is to provide activity during therapy sessions which requires the active participation of the children (as far as they are able) to improve motor skills and motor planning abilities. This is often best accomplished by working jointly with other professionals.

A good example of this approach is our work with Alex. Whilst he sits on a suspended swing, moving in a regular pattern of linear movement, a colleague who is a speech and language therapist works on basic sound systems. Over time, we observe an increase in Alex's eye-contact, he begins to articulate some basic sounds, and then slowly he begins to interact. The movement input of the swing appears to have assisted Alex in being available for communication in engaging with his environment. Working jointly with another professional like this enables a sharing of ideas and an opportunity to work with a child when he or she is sensorily available to do so.

A typically developing child provides his brain with necessary sensory experiences through play. He jumps a little higher on the trampoline, swings head down lying over a swing, mixes the jam into his rice pudding with his fingers. Such experiences provide the brain with sensory information. They help the brain to respond in a meaningful manner to each sensory input. Unfortunately, as the risk of litigation invades our society, our school playgrounds, parks and playgrounds have become places of limited sensory experience. Roundabouts have been removed, slides made smaller and swing chains shortened. Children are left to seek out the sensory experiences they need in other, less appropriate, ways. An eight-year-old boy in one of the schools in which I work was found riding his bike down the stairs in an effort to provide himself with vestibular/movement input! Children need to develop basic sensori-motor foundations on which to build the higher-level abilities involved in language and cognitive development.

Often what is interpreted by adults as misbehaviour is the child's attempt at meeting his or her own central nervous system needs. The child may merely need adult assistance to find a more appropriate way of meeting that specific sensory need.

As a therapist of Sensory Integration, I choose activities for the child that provide controlled sensory input. From an outsider's point of view, the child is merely playing. From a Sensory Integration point of view, the child is helped to manage negative sensory responses and make adaptive responses that help to organise the central nervous system. The therapist assists the child to do this and to participate as actively as he or she is able.

Therapy offers many movement and sensory experiences. However, such experiences need to be carefully monitored. Certain movement/vestibular inputs can be very powerful. The effect may not become evident until after the child has left the therapy room. Repeated observation and assessment allows the therapist to recognise when a child is becoming sensorily overloaded. Sensory overload can occur quickly and easily in central nervous systems that have difficulty integrating input. The therapist needs to teach parents, carers and teachers to recognise the signs of imminent sensory overload and to know what action to take. James's breathing rate was seen to increase when he rotated on a tyre swing. He became hot, red and very loud. The swing was stopped. He was encouraged to retire to a den within the room to allow his central nervous system to reorganise and calm.

These examples, then, give ideas about how the insights offered to us by Sensory Integration Theory can be developed into intervention strategies. The key element that is needed for such intervention is an awareness of how significant our sensory systems are to our behaviour.

Environments and sensory responses

One other element that Sensory Integration Theory teaches us is to be aware of the environment within which people are functioning. Environments can either assist our functioning or interfere with it. By identifying and changing aspects of the environment that are problematic, we can dramatically improve our levels of calmness and thus effectiveness in the world – for example, a dimmer switch fitted to the lights can assist an individual with visual sensitivity.

I am trying to write this section sitting at the kitchen table at home. It is the end of the summer holidays and the house is full of students who are not working, nor have any desire to do so! The kitchen, during the day, has slowly filled with clutter. Cups, glasses, plates and 'things' now overwhelm the work surfaces around me. People walk in and out. Snippets of conversation occur around me. My neighbour has decided to mow the lawn.

I am now aware that the combination of visual clutter, noise and movement around me is creating sensory disorganisation. My thought processes are slowing. I am feeling irritated. Even my ability to put the letters in the correct order in a word is compromised. The environment I find myself in is not conducive to the task in hand. *I cannot get on with writing this chapter!* The environment that a person is in always impacts directly upon his or her behaviour, stress levels and emotional state.

For an individual with a disordered sensory integration, a particular environment may evoke painful or negative behavioural responses that result in the individual self-harming or harming others. Visual, auditory, olfactory, tactile and movement/vestibular sensations within a specific environment can have a positive or negative impact upon an individual's sensory organisation. The colour of the room, the background noise, the floor covering, the surrounding scents and odours, the opportunities to move or not, all have a sensory impact.

I am always struck by the impact of environments when I am asked to work with children in schools. For example, I was recently invited to work with Jay, a young man on the autistic spectrum, who attended a special school. Previous assessments had shown that Jay was hypersensitive to noise and that he coped with this sensitivity through 'tactile defensiveness'. During the period when I was visiting his classroom, a young girl in the class started to wail and then to scream. Another child joined in, outside the window. The school lawns were also being cut by a large, sit-on mower. Adults started to raise their voices in an effort to try to overcome the noise makers.

Jay coped with all this stimulation by putting his hands over his ears and withdrawing under a table. This meant, though, that Jay was not part of the group any more, so two adults approached Jay's space under the table, and reached in to pull him out of it. He reacted to this threat by hitting out, and then by banging his head repeatedly against the table. In short, Jay's environment had produced sensory disorganisation for him and, eventually, sensory meltdown. Jay was now in 'survival' mode, unable actively to participate in any educational or constructive interaction with adults.

Other schools with which I work ensure that their staff receive regular training in Sensory Integration Theory. In one school, they have created a safe place where specific students can retire to when becoming sensorily disorganised and overwhelmed. The 'safe place' in this case is a throw-up tent in the corner of a room, containing ear-defenders, sunglasses and a weighted blanket.

Adam has severe ADHD and learning difficulties and is on the autistic spectrum. Adam can easily become overwhelmed by noise, movement, smells and touch. Unable to filter out unimportant sensory information, he can quickly become 'sensory full'. In this school, staff monitor Adam's behaviour. When they see him becoming sweaty, loud and restless, he is encouraged, with a favourite book and a favourite member of staff, to retire to the tent. There, he puts on the sunglasses, snuggles under the weighted blanket and begins to enjoy a calming story. Staff report that because Adam rarely hits sensory overload these days, they find he is more cooperative throughout the school day. His school work has shown noticeable improvement. His social interaction skills are also such that he can now sit at a table with other children and work alongside them.

Harriet, whom we have met before, has an intense need for movement in order to integrate her senses and, in particular, to reduce her sensitivity to auditory stimulation. If Harriet actively plays for at least 45 minutes outside on the equipment in her garden (whatever the weather!), she is calm and cooperative at bed-time. Her home environment is now geared towards periods of active play, and Harriet is now able to cope with the tasks of getting dressed, sitting to eat, and allowing her mum to apply sun cream. When Harriet's environment and Harriet's day are geared to movement and movement sensation, then we have found that her eye-contact increases, cooperative play occurs, and she expresses words and sounds that previously she did not. Harriet is more available for communication and to engage with her environment.

When you are unable to organise the sensations coming into your body, the world appears a confusing, threatening place. In contrast, if the environments in which you spend your time correspond to your sensory needs, then your central nervous system will receive positive sensory inputs that will organise and calm, resulting in engagement, communication and availability for learning. When staff provide activities that allow for central nervous system reorganisation throughout the day it enables the children in their care to participate in their environment more effectively and certainly to the best of their ability.

Providing such activities requires that carers observe an individual's style of functioning in different settings, with different people, at different times. Such observation ensures that each individual's unique pattern of sensory processing is understood. We can then adapt environments accordingly and provide individuals with the sensory input their central nervous systems need. This assists not only those individuals, but it assists those caring for them, for in reducing anxiety levels, stubbornness, explosive behaviours and withdrawal also decrease. Their communication abilities and their capacity to learn begin to improve quite markedly.

Conclusion

This chapter was not easy to write. It created a whole range of sensory needs for me along the way – numerous biscuits, cups of tea and visits to the gym! I hope that it helps to fulfil part of Dr A. Jean Ayres's mission in life. That mission was to spread the word regarding Sensory Integration

Theory, educating parents, carers and other professionals about the powerful insights it offers us. Such insights apply to all the domains discussed in this book – infants, autism, severe neglect, deafblindness, dementia – even where the authors have not considered sensory issues in their chapters.

Through the understanding that Sensory Integration Theory affords us, we can begin to look at other people in more thoughtful, respectful ways. We can begin to interpret their behaviours as a means of survival, rather than calculated sabotage! Through our own understanding, we become able to improve the experiences of others, helping them to lead calmer, more fulfilling lives.

References

Ayres, A.J. (1979) *Sensory Integration and the Child.* Los Angeles, CA: Western Psychological Services.

Ayres, A.J. (1989) *Sensory Integration and Praxis Test (SIPT).* Los Angeles, CA: Western Psychological Services.

Baraneck, G.T. (1999) 'Autism during infancy: A retrospective video analysis of sensory-motor and social behaviors at 9–12 months of age.' *Journal of Autism and Developmental Disorders 29,* 213–224.

Cooper, J., Majnemer, A., Rosenblatt, B. and Birnbaum, R. (1995) 'The determination of sensory deficits in children with hemiplegic cerebral palsy.' *Journal of Child Neurology 10,* 300–309.

Dawson, G. and Adams, A. (1984) 'Imitation and social responsiveness in autistic children.' *Journal of Abnormal Child Psychology 12,* 209–226.

Dunn, W. (1999) *Sensory Profile.* San Antonio, TX: The Psychological Corporation (www.sensoryprofile.com).

Greenspan, S.I. and Wieder, S. (1997) 'Developmental patterns and outcomes in infants and children with disorders in relating and communicating: A chart review of 200 cases of children with autistic spectrum diagnoses.' *Journal of Developmental and Learning Disorders 1,* 87–141.

Lesny, I., Stehlik, A., Tomasek, J., Tomankova, A. and Havlicek I. (1993) 'Sensory disorders in cerebral palsy: Two-point discrimination.' *Developmental Medicine and Child Neurology 35,* 402–405.

Osterling, J. and Dawson, G. (1994) 'Early recognition of children with autism: A study of first birthday home videotapes.' *Journal of Autism and Developmental Disorders 24,* 247–257.

Williams, D. (1998) *Like Colour to the Blind: Soul Searching and Soul Finding.* London: Jessica Kingsley Publishers.

Williams, M.S. and Shellenberger, S. (1994) 'The Alert Program for self-regulation.' *American Occupational Therapy Association, Sensory Integration Special Interest Section Newsletter,* 17, 1–3.

CHAPTER 11

INTENSIVE INTERACTION: GETTING IN TOUCH WITH A CHILD WITH SEVERE AUTISM

Phoebe Caldwell

My name is Phoebe Caldwell and I am a practitioner who has been working with people with Autistic Spectrum Disorder and severe learning disabilities for 35 years. Around 15 years ago, I held a Joseph Rowntree Research Fellowship for four years. My supervisor was a psychologist called Geraint Ephraim. It was he who introduced the technique that uses people's own body language to build up a non-verbal way of communicating with them, now known as Intensive Interaction.

This chapter is an individual study of using this approach with an eight-year-old child who has extremely severe autism. It should be noted that the child in question is from a European country and English is not part of his life. I mention this because, in our multicultural society, Intensive Interaction can be used independently of the child's first language.

In the course of practice I work with individuals who are often extremely disturbed and present difficult management problems. I also teach those who support them, an audience that includes psychologists, managers, therapists, support workers and, just as vital (since the information they receive is often sketchy), parent groups. I have written a number of books, and taken part in several training videos, on the subject of communication with non-verbal or semi-verbal individuals (Caldwell 2000, 2002, 2004, 2005, 2006). My latest book is entitled *From Isolation to Intimacy* (2007), and a handbook for using Intensive Interaction with children and adults on the autistic spectrum is currently in the process of publication, entitled *Using Intensive Interaction and Sensory Integration: A Handbook for those who Support People with Severe Autism.*

What I should like to do in this chapter is look for the answers to three questions. What is Intensive Interaction? What does it feel like to be a child with Autistic Spectrum Disorder? And finally, how does Intensive Interaction help us to get in touch with such a child?

Intensive Interaction

Intensive Interaction is the name of an approach that uses body language to communicate with people whom we find it difficult to reach. Although it can be used effectively with some people who have speech, most of the partners with whom Intensive Interaction practitioners work are non-verbal. Some have severe or profound learning disabilities.

Intensive Interaction is particularly effective in establishing emotional engagement with people who have very severe Autistic Spectrum Disorder and are locked into an inner world, either focusing on one of their own body sensations or rhythms, or fixating on a sensory stimulus hijacked from an object or activity from the world outside. They then use the feedback they derive from this activity to supply the brain with the particular sensation which gives them a point of focus. In the middle of sensory chaos it provides them with coherence. When we use Intensive Interaction with them, our aim is to tap into our partners' internal conversation and shift their attention from solitary self stimulation to shared activity. What they were doing by themselves becomes the basis of a dialogue. In sensory terms, we can talk to each other.

As other authors in this book discuss (e.g. in Chapters 4 and 7), the basis of Intensive Interaction is observation and imitation, but both these terms are misleading in that they limit the scope of what such an approach has to offer. To begin with, 'observation' implies independent witness, a space that distances observer from observed (I stand aside and watch what you do). This is not how I would describe the way that I practise. My priority is 'attention', not just to what my partners are doing, but also to *how* they are doing it, since this tells me how they are feeling. A speech therapist I worked with defined this quality as 'intimate attention'. In order to build in empathy to my responses, I need to use all my senses to tune in to the affective quality of their activity. I need to feel what *they* feel in *my* own bones. First of all I empty myself and place myself entirely at my partner's disposal.

Sometimes our partners are listening to an activity as slight as their own breathing rhythm. The brain is telling the body to breathe in and the body is sending feedback in the form of sensation, telling the brain that it has done this. As practitioners, we need to tune in to this feedback. This is the sensation that has significance for their brain, one that it recognises as non-threatening. We can use this to infiltrate our partner's brain–body conversation.

One of the commonest ways that people with autism carry on these self-stimulatory behaviours is to scratch their hands in one way or another. The brain says 'scratch' to the thumb or fingers and gets back a specific sensation. It may be quite hard to spot this if our partner's hands are curled up into a fist or hidden under her arms. But once we recognize how she is talking to herself we can answer this in a number of ways. We can sit near her and copy what she is doing, giving her a visual response. Or we can scratch the movement on a chair or rough material so that she hears a related rhythm. Alternatively, and if she will allow us, we can use touch, making a scratching movement on her shoulder or foot or wherever she may find touch acceptable. We will probably find that one mode is more effective than another, so we need to monitor our partner's responses with total attention. What effect does it have if I do exactly the same as she does, and what difference is there if I do it slightly differently from the way she is doing it? It should be noted that if we are using touch it needs to be part of a management strategy, outlining for staff exactly what is and is not acceptable. An anxiety about touch exists within today's society, which needs to be acknowledged, but it should also be realised that there are some people on the autistic spectrum who are unable to respond to visual or auditory stimuli and for whom touch, particularly deep touch which stimulates the proprioceptive system, may be the only way we can get through to them. This point is one that Jane Horwood explores in more detail in Chapter 10, on Sensory Integration.

Most of the people I am asked to see are severely disturbed and difficult to engage. An example: a child with very severe behavioural disturbance swishes her leg over a waterbed. I scratch the wood-chip wallpaper in time to her movement. She then smacks her leg on the waterbed she is lying on. I bang the wall. She bounces the waterbed. I bounce her back, at first in the same rhythm and then use a different rhythm. This is a joke: her brain is expecting one response but gets a related but different one. She laughs. She leads as we expand the range of her games, ending up piling her feet and my hands alternately, a version she introduces of the child's game, 'One potato, two potatoes, three potatoes, four...'

Some people will say that they feel stupid using such 'childish' activities – and if our partners are grown up, to do so is disrespectful to the adult they now are. This argument is mistaken. It is the outcome of our failure to recognise the actual sensory reality experienced by our partner and to appreciate that this differs from our own. This argument fails to ask what it is in our partner's sensory perception of his or her environment that has meaning for his or her brain, making the erroneous assumption that the two of us are perceiving the reality we share in the same way. Just because I feel, see and hear the world around me in one way, it is incorrect to assume your sensory experience of the world to be the same. From here, is easy to fall into the trap of basing not only our strategies on such a false premise but also our behavioural judgements. A child who kicks the walls may be thought to be 'naughty' when – because he sees it as moving – he is actually trying to sort out where he is in relation to it.

In practice, using a person's body language is not difficult since it is already part of the way we all communicate with each other. We are monitoring each other's bodies all the time. Like any conversation, we respond to whatever is passing between us at the time. We take turns, give each other time, pick up on any new initiatives and introduce new material ourselves. But in using Intensive Interaction, it is important that any new material introduced into the conversation be offered within the context of the existing theme. It should not stray so far that the connection becomes blurred.

The use of body language in this way could be called 'imitation', although I think this term too limited. Once again, it implies a distance between the two partners, and an objectification, where one partner simply performs the same action that the other partner has just performed. This is not what I am doing when using Intensive Interaction. Rather, I am responding to the person I am talking to, using his or her body language.

More importantly, this process of imitation (if one wishes to call it that) is in itself only a starting point, a way of capturing attention, a door to enter the inner world of our partners. It is not the endpoint. The destinations are a matter for mutual negotiation and are sometimes amazing.

In this context I want to introduce the story of Davy, a small boy who I have chosen to talk about because the work that I and his teachers have done with him illustrates how observation and use of a person's body language can reach through to them even when their behaviour is extremely

complex and distressed. It also gives expression to the astonishing inge-
nuity of a non-verbal child in finding a way to express how he feels.

I visited Davy twice, the first time to introduce his teachers to Intensive Interaction and the second time to see the progress which had been
made. Between the first and second visit there was a gap of eight months
but since Davy had been seriously ill and in hospital, by the time of the
second visit his teachers had been using Intensive Interaction with him
for approximately three months.

Davy: A history

Davy is eight years old. He has very severe Autistic Spectrum Disorder.
When he started school his behaviour was extremely distressed and he
spent much of his time screaming and throwing himself about. It became
clear that he was unable to cope with the sensory overload he was experiencing in a class with other children. He was moved to his own room. He
now has two teachers with him all the time. The TEACCH (Treatment
and Education of Autistic and Related Communication Handicapped
Children) method (which is now commonly used to institute greater
structure and predictability within the lives of individuals with autism) is
used to provide him with an ordered timetable, and he has benefited from
a structured environment and schedule.

However, Davy still lives in a world on his own. He makes little
eye-contact. He does make sounds but clearly does not know how to use
these for communication. These become louder noises when he is upset,
and he throws tantrums and screams. He has shown some improvement
since he first arrived and was able to move to a separate classroom. His
distressed behaviour is now intermittent rather than continuous but nevertheless can be very severe.

When Davy walks down the passage he drags his hand along the
wall. He has an unusual fixation in that he is totally locked into the words
he sees on television. His favourite occupation is to spell these out in
Play-doh on his desk, even putting in the most minute details of the font.
For example he will spell out, 'Walt Disney' and peer at it intently. The
interest he displays in this activity contrasts with the way that he relates to
his 'educational' programme of tabletop puzzles, putting together nuts
and bolts and completing puzzles. He does these apparently because they
are an activity he knows he has to do but completes without interest. On
the other hand, when he is motivated, he can pick up a camera lens and fit

it over the cap without any difficulty, a similar task, but one that has meaning for him when he is saying to us that he does not wish to be filmed.

Davy needs to know what is happening in his schedule. Problems arise when there is a gap between activities and when he cannot immediately see what is coming next. His school's present strategy for managing this need is to give him the token that symbolises his name. He then goes to the desk in the passage outside the room and fetches the picture of his next activity. If this does not go smoothly, however, he loses track and becomes distraught. The activities need to be close at hand. He shows no self-motivation. When his teacher puts out her hand he gives her the bits to complete. When he gets stuck he screeches. To some extent he uses the PECS (Picture Exchange Communication System) system (i.e. reference cards allowing individuals to make requests of others) that he has been taught in the same disinterested way. He recognises the pictures on the cards and knows what to do with them but it is as if the process is merely something he has to do to get what he wants. He does it without any interest in personal interaction. To summarise, Davy is very closed off indeed, living in his own world and keeping the external sensory chaos at bay.

One of the trigger points for Davy's distress has been getting him in from playtime, to the point at which this is setting off such violent distress that his teachers are discussing whether it would be better to suspend taking him outside.

The question we need to answer in order to help Davy is: out of all the environmental and internal turmoil that he is experiencing, which sensory stimuli have meaning for his brain? Which particular feedback is he using to maintain coherence and give himself some idea of what is going on around him?

Using Intensive Interaction with Davy

FIRST VISIT

What is very clear is the extreme degree of sensory confusion that Davy experiences. However, in my first meeting with him I am struck by the way he orientates himself vis-à-vis the wall by dragging his finger along the surface: he appears to be giving himself tactile stimulus. This fingertip sensation is how he maintains coherence, a sense of what he is doing. One of his former teachers tells me that he can sometimes be calmed by squeezing his shoulders firmly like kneading dough, giving him proprioceptive feedback.

The most obvious way to talk to Davy through his body language is to answer the sounds he makes. I try this, but responding to these does not seem to reach through to his inner world. He gives no sign that my initiatives mean anything to him. However, when he is outside he gets astride a rocker. At this stage I introduce sounds which coincide with the rhythm of his bumps, my voice tuned into his sounds but moving up and down coincident with his movements. His teachers join in. Davy's facial language alters and he begins to look round for the source of these sounds – his sounds but not his sounds – referring back with interest and looking from myself to his two teachers to see if we would do it again. He smiles at us, turning from one to another. We share his pleasure. There is good eye-contact. Linking his sounds with the contingent see-saw bang of the rocker as it hits the ground introduces an element of surprise that has been sufficient to capture the attention of his brain. Taking this together with his use of tactile stimulus to know what he is doing when he walks down the passage, I suggest that while his visual and auditory processing easily become overloaded, his ability to process tactile and proprioceptive sensations is less vulnerable. When his attention is switched from his inner world by a stimulus that is significant for his brain, he is able to make sense of relevant sounds. He begins to take even more notice of his sounds when he is being held and rocked.

The relative stability of his proprioceptive sense is further suggested when we work on the problems he experiences in coming back into his classroom at the end of breaktime. Davy is used to being left to his own devices outside and it is difficult to persuade him to come in. He is so locked into his own world that when he is shown the PECS card that tells him it is time to come in, he does not appear to see it.

Remembering that he is apparently more sensitive to touch than visual clues, using it to orientate himself, I suggest that we use his Play-doh pot as an object of reference so that he can feel it as well as see it. He gets up quickly and comes in but again stops when he is halfway across the metal ramp. Although he starts off towards his classroom, he quickly loses track of what he is doing and lies down and refuses to come any further. He does not respond to persuasion. At this point the practice has been to lift him up and carry him in. He becomes extremely upset. Once he is upset he is completely distraught and extremely difficult to calm.

I suggest we let him lie and try using touch to refocus him. Every time he makes a sound I nudge his foot. After a short while he kneels up and holds the metal guardrail. I put my hands outside and play with his fingers. He puts his nose against the wire and I press it *when he makes a sound*. Linking my pressure to his sound is very important in reaching through to Davy. He gets on his hands and knees, his hand splayed out against the grating. I run my pen round it making a rough sound and vibration on the metal. He keeps moving his hand so I will repeat this. Then he stands up and walks to the classroom by himself! We have had a breakthrough. His teachers are delighted.

At breaktime on the second day Davy is not particularly interested in the sounds we make when he is on the rocker – but he is entranced by the sound of a nearby tractor engine. This suggests to me that he may hear low sounds better than high ones. He also stops and looks up intently when I bang my feet heavily on the metal stair. We encourage him on to the tyre swing, as he enjoys big swings on it. I slow him down to stop and then swing him very gently side to side, making *contingent* low sounds like the tractor. Although he is not answering my sounds he becomes very thoughtful and listens intently. Then he begins to respond by wriggling his feet when he wants more. I wriggle my hands in answer and swing him again.

When it is time for Davy to return to his class we give him the Play-doh tub – but this time it is filled to the brim with Play-doh to make it feel heavy. The added weight should keep his proprioceptive system more active. He carries it straight in through the door without stopping, even though it means breaking off an activity he is really enjoying. It is now clear that what Davy needs to inform him is proprioceptive stimulus. When he is getting this he knows what he is doing and he is able to relate to his surroundings – and he is able to do this in a way that has not previously been possible.

Once inside, Davy plays with his dough. As usual, he makes his letters in a single colour. I ask his teacher to make the same letters, but in another colour. During this time Davy is totally self-absorbed. He makes a new shape which looks like a twisted candle on a mount with three little nodules on the top. Later he puts one in his mouth and uses it as a 'pipe' for smoking. I assume this is something he has seen on TV.

I want to join in so I sit beside Davy and take some of his dough. At first he grabs it back but becomes more tolerant and eventually allows me to make one of his shapes and stand it close to his. He keeps on referring back to my object to see what I am doing. At this stage my object certainly has meaning for him in respect of comparison with his. He is not, however, interested in me as a person.

The next day Davy makes a pirate boat he has seen on TV. This is an extremely accurate representation with all its details: masts, flag and oar. It does have real meaning for him, since at the end he quite deliberately pokes a hole in the side with his finger and then scrunches it up. He is telling us the story that he saw on television – that the ship has been sunk. The next day he builds his ship again and his teacher builds one at the same time, in a different colour. He keeps checking to see what she is doing and smiling.

We move on to letters, which Davy makes from Play-doh. He spells 'Walt Disney', which I again assume he has previously seen on TV.

I decide to try something novel – spelling out a word that Davy has not introduced but which would be meaningful to him. I decide to use his name, so I spell out 'Davy'. He grabs the letter from me and scrunches them up. Instead, I add a letter to the front of the word he is making. I am teasing him just a bit. At first Davy pushes my letter away, but then he begins to enjoy the joke and he smiles – at me. This is a landmark moment. I am no longer the object. Davy is becoming interested in me as a person. Given our earlier successes with constructing figures and letters that he has seen on TV, it occurs to me that he might be more interested in writing out 'Davy' in Play-doh if it were done in the orientation he is used to seeing on TV. That is, I decide to try displaying the letters in a vertical fashion, rather than the more standard horizontal orientation we have been using. So we stick a metal board to the wall and I put up the magnetic letters D, A, V, and Y. Davy first takes the letters away, but then he spells out 'Davy' on the board by himself. Our reorienting of the letters has proven successful; he is engaged in the task.

Later, Davy's teacher is using pens and paper with him, drawing circles. I suggest she write 'Davy', which she does. Davy holds her hand for a bit while she draws letters and then indicates for her to repeat the word. She does this several times and then writes 'Bill', his father's name. He spends considerable time comparing the two words and appears to be really thinking about what he is seeing. We put them up on the board in front of him.

SECOND VISIT (AFTER THREE MONTHS OF INTENSIVE INTERACTION)

Davy's teachers have been working very hard with him using his body language to interact with him. He has clearly changed: he is much happier and less inclined to outbursts of disturbed behaviour. When he does have one of these, using firm pressure on his shoulders is normally effective in calming him.

His workstation is now screened more effectively so that he is getting fewer extraneous stimuli. His number and colour flash cards are on the wall (vertical as seen on TV) and he relates to these very well. These changes make it easier for him to relate to whatever stimuli he is presented with.

At one point, Davy begins to make a necklace from his construction kit, fitting the pieces together carefully and, when it is complete, placing it round his neck. His teacher makes use of one of the more orthodox aspects of Intensive Interaction based on imitation. She makes an identical one. The following day, Davy has another teacher and he makes necklaces with her also, leaning over to adjust a piece of hers so that, like his, it is symmetrical. When she adds an extra piece, Davy dives into his box and adds an identical one to his. This goes on for some time, she copying him and he copying her. He is smiling at her. On the third day I am absent but meet his teacher in the afternoon. She greets me, saying: 'You'll never guess what Davy did today. He made his necklace and I made an identical one. When we had both finished he took a few more pieces out of his box and joined our necklaces together. His face was radiant.'

WHAT DIFFERENCE DOES USING INTENSIVE INTERACTION MAKE TO DAVY'S LIFE EXPERIENCE?

When he is calm, Davy has three easily identifiable states. In the first, he has no connection with the world around him; he is lost in his inner world. We saw the second when he was on the swing. I stopped it swinging backwards and forwards and swung it very gently sideways. He became very attentive to what was clearly a novel sensation for him. At the same time this did not increase his interactivity. He was far too interested in the feeling itself. The third state can only be described as 'switched on'. He is sharing pleasure with his communication partner. We need to be aware of these three states when we are interacting with him. What is it exactly that grabs and holds Davy's attention so that its direction becomes interpersonal?

When I practise Intensive Interaction, it helps to be well embodied, to know what I am feeling. As Davy runs his hand along the rough wall, I am so aware of this that, without putting out my hand, I also feel its roughness in my fingertips. The 'mirror neurons' in my brain, which science has discovered so much about during the last decade (e.g. Ramachandran and Oberman 2006; Rizzolatti *et al.* 1995), recognize a sensation that is part of my stored memory, playing it back as a scratchy feeling through my flesh. I am in tune with the way that Davy is using touch to maintain coherence. This is a stimulus he relies on to know what he is doing. And it is not only touch that he uses but also proprioceptive sensation, that is, internal feelings in his muscles and joints. I need to remain in touch with this sensation myself, in order to help Davy.

When his sounds (which he does not attend to) are linked to his movements (which do have meaning for him), one is effectively drawing his own attention to his sounds. His teacher has dressed him to go out. He is sitting on a chair pushing his feet against the shoe locker in a rhythmic way. She tunes his sounds into his rhythm and he smiles quietly at her with good eye-contact. And on the rocker, Davy is entranced when we put his sounds together with the bumps he is giving himself.

When Davy loses his sense of what is happening he lies on the ground. It is the safest place. Gunilla Gerland (1996) describes this loss of a meaningful picture of the world round her in her book *A Real Person*, giving us a powerful insight into what it feels like to be on the autistic spectrum. When she 'lost coherence' and could not work out what was happening, she had no idea where her feet were, or where 'up' and 'down' had gone. If Davy has laid down on the ground to reorient himself because his brain is overloaded, and then we forcibly pick him up, in order to move him inside, Davy's sensory processing system breaks up completely. He goes into 'fragmentation', a state that Ramachandran terms an 'autonomic storm' (Ramachandran and Oberman 2006). Alternatively (using the insight we have already gained), if we offer him a heavy weight to carry (e.g. a bucket of Play-doh), he can make sense of this. It gives him a point of focus which helps to carry him through the task of coming in from the playground into his classroom.

It is more difficult to work out exactly what processes are going on in Davy's brain when he his makes his drawings and models reproducing what he sees on TV. It is clear that he sees images with extraordinary detail. He collects words and pictures. Following his watching of the film 'Madagascar', he both models and draws a giraffe, a lion and a zebra, clearly distinguishable from each other. He fixates on them with deep intensity, all his senses concentrating on them, and then suddenly breaks them up. One might almost say he attacks and destroys them, just as he earlier sank his boat. Such stability as he derives from his fixation is reduced to chaos. Whether purposefully or not, Davy is showing us the autonomic storm that periodically goes on inside his head.

However, what has also become very clear is that Davy loves interaction with people – when it is presented in a mode that is part of his repertoire and therefore does not add to his sensory confusion. Under these conditions he visibly relaxes. And when he is relaxed he is able to accomplish a number of things that are at variance with the expectations suggested by research into autism.

For example, current research indicates that people on the autistic spectrum are unable to imitate the actions of other people. A recent explanation of this 'failure' is that their mirror neurons are not firing in the same way as those of people not on the spectrum. This explains their difficulty in relating to other people (Baron-Cohen, Leslie and Frith 1985). But contrary to this claim, Davy both imitates and relates extremely well *when we use the mode of communication that is part of his repertoire.* He can copy exactly what is being offered to him. So it seems logical to assume that his mirror neurons are firing normally under these user-friendly conditions. To say that the mirror neurons are deficient in people with autism is like saying that we cannot start a car when we have flooded the engine. There is nothing wrong with the motor, rather it is our practice that is at fault.

Recent investigations suggest that when 'imitation' (or approaches based on imitation) is used with children or adults who are on the autistic spectrum, their social responsiveness improves. Chapters 4 and 6 demonstrate this effect. So also does Nadel's work in France (e.g. Nadel *et al.* 2000; Nadel and Pezé 1993), including several later studies that have followed up this work, which show that even very brief periods of imitation are sufficient to dramatically increase autistic children's interest in another person (Escalona *et al.* 2002; Field *et al.* 2001; Heimann, Laberg and Nordøen 2006). Ingersoll, based in the US, has obtained similar findings using a technique that she calls Reciprocal Imitation Training (Ingersoll and Schreibman 2006). And in other work I am carrying out with colleagues (Zeedyk, Caldwell and Davies 2007), we have been using frame by frame analyses of video material to try to code in detail the growth of interpersonal engagement that occurs with the use of Intensive Interaction. We have looked at four variables – eye gaze, proximity, orientation to partner and positive emotion – and have been able to show, quantitatively, the degree to which each of these behaviours increases over the course of a session of Intensive Interaction.

However broken down, study after study shows the same pattern – that although the time taken to effect change may differ (in some cases the time-line is short, in others it takes longer), the sequence is the same: imitation is accompanied by an increase in intimacy.

His teacher's use of Intensive Interaction results not just in an improvement in Davy's behaviour. There is a change in his ability to relate to the world around him and to engage with people. He now knows that his teachers will take his initiatives and attempts to communicate seriously and will value his initiatives as they are. The reduction in the amount of his disturbed outbursts indicates clearly that he no longer finds his environment the terrifying place that it was for him before.

I should emphasise that the story of Davy is not a one-off. The aim of my books has been to describe this process, again and again, in regard to the many new people I meet in the course of my work. It is amazing to see our partners come to life. The change in alertness, capacity to relate and general body language is so evident that people who come in after interactions will comment on the difference. They are both more relaxed and more alert. Time and again, the parents of children I have worked with say that at last they have happy children. A sister was so moved by the change realised in her brother that she said, 'I want to go out and teach everybody how to do this!' Once the brain is not being overloaded by unprocessed images and sounds, the capacity to interact is intact.

We are now able to lift our partners out of their inner world where they are so frightened. Apart from being able to have fun with our partners, now that we have found ways of getting in touch with them, we can use their sounds and movements 'bilingually', so that we cannot only gain their attention but also hold it when we speak in 'our own language', effectively 'gift-wrapping' the bits they may find scary. For example, a child who is frightened in shops can be constantly reassured and refocused into safety by hearing her partner make 'her sounds'. Like the 'cats-eyes' in the road that indicate where it is safe to drive, these sounds become markers which tell the child where it is safe to go.

So, in spite of Davy being one of the most severely affected children on the autistic spectrum I have met, when we use Intensive Interaction with him, Davy can both imitate and relate. He is not only very good at copying but also, in a moment that has to be described as inspired, he uses this capacity to show his teacher how close he feels to her, by joining up their necklaces. His non-verbal capacity to express emotional engagement is astonishing and he relishes her response. His eye-contact improves. He is interested in his teacher's response and refers back to her. Although he cannot speak words, his actions speak volumes.

As well as using our partner's language to improve communication, we must listen to what they tell us. Using Intensive Interaction is not something we do *to* our partners. At its best, it is about exchange, about respect, about learning from each other and learning to value what is important to them – and so showing them how valuable they are, giving them a sense of their intrinsic worth as people.

ACKNOWLEDGEMENTS

I should like to thank to Davy's headmaster and his parents for permission to use material arising from interactive sessions at Davy's school, and also to express my admiration for his teachers and the enthusiasm which they have brought to the processes of Intensive Interaction.

References

Baron-Cohen, S., Leslie, A.M. and Frith, U. (1985) 'Does the autistic child have a theory of mind?' *Cognition 21*, 37–46.

Caldwell, P. (2000) *You Don't Know What It's Like: Finding Ways of Building Relationships with People with Severe Learning Disabilities, Autistic Spectrum Disorder and Other Impairments.* Brighton: Pavilion Publishing.

Caldwell, P. (2002) *Learning the Language: Building Relationships with People with Severe Learning Disability, Autistic Spectrum Disorder and Other Challenging Behaviours.* Brighton: Pavilion Publishing.

Caldwell, P. (2004) *Crossing the Minefield: Establishing Safe Passage through the Sensory Chaos of Austistic Spectrum Disorder.* Brighton: Pavilion Publishing.

Caldwell, P. (2005) *Creative Conversations: Communicating with People with Profound and Multiple Learning Disabilities.* Brighton: Pavilion Publishing.

Caldwell, P. (2006) *Finding You, Finding Me: Using Intensive Interaction to Get in Touch with People whose Severe Learning Disabilities are Combined with Autistic Spectrum Disorder.* London: Jessica Kingsley Publishers.

Caldwell, P. (2007) *From Isolation to Intimacy: Making Friends Without Words.* London: Jessica Kingsley Publishers.

Escalona, A., Field, T., Nadel, J. and Lundy, B. (2002) 'Brief report: Imitation effects on children with autism.' *Journal of Autism and Developmental Disorders 32*, 141–144.

Field, T., Field, T., Sanders, C. and Nadel, J. (2001) 'Children with autism display more social behaviors after repeated imitation sessions.' *Autism 5*, 3, 317–323.

Gerland, G. (1996) *A Real Person.* London: Souvenir Press.

Heimann, M., Laberg, K.E. and Nordøen, B. (2006) 'Imitative interaction increases social interest and elicited imitation in non-verbal children with autism.' *Infant and Child Development 15,* 297–309.

Ingersoll, B. and Schreibman, L. (2006) 'Teaching reciprocal imitation skills to young children with autism using a naturalistic behavioral approach: Effects on language, pretend play, and joint attention.' *Journal of Autism and Developmental Disorders 36,* 487–505.

Nadel, J., Croué, S., Mattlinger, M.-J., Canet, P., Hudelot, C., Lecuyer, C. and Martini, M. (2000) 'Do children with autism have expectancies about the social behaviour of unfamiliar people?' *Autism 4,* 133–145.

Nadel, J. and Pezé, A. (1993) 'What makes immediate imitation communicative in toddlers and autistic children?' In J. Nadel and L. Camaioni (eds) *New Perspectives in Early Communicative Development.* London: Routledge.

Ramachandran, V.S. and Oberman, L.M. (2006) 'Broken mirrors: A theory of autism.' *Scientific American 295* (November), 39–45.

Rizzolatti, G., Camarda, R., Gallese, V. and Fogassik L. (1995) 'Premotor cortex and the recognition of motor actions.' *Cognitive Brain Research 3,* 131–141.

Zeedyk, M.S., Caldwell, P. and Davies, C.E. (2007) 'Imitation promotes social engagement in adults with severe autism and learning disabilities.' Submitted to *Journal of Autism and Developmental Disorders.*

THE CONTRIBUTORS

Arlene J. Astell is a Lecturer in Psychology based in the Dementia Research Group at the University of St Andrews. She can be contacted on aja3@st-and.ac.uk.

Naomi Betts graduated from the University of Dundee in 2007 with an Honours degree in psychology, having carried out analyses described in Chapter 6 as part of her final year research dissertation.

Phoebe Caldwell is an independent practitioner of Intensive Interaction, based in Lancashire. She can be contacted on phoebecaldwell@btopenworld.com.

Pete Coia is the Principal Clinical Psychologist for Wakefield and Pontefract Learning Disability Psychology Service. He can be contacted on pete.coia@swyt.nhs.uk.

Clifford E. Davies is an Honorary Lecturer in Psychology, in the School of Psychology at the University of St Andrews. Information relevant to Chapter 6 can be obtained from either the first or second author, on cliff.davies@hotmail.co.uk or m.s.zeedyk@dundee.ac.uk.

Maggie P. Ellis is currently a PhD student within the Dementia Research Group, based in the School of Psychology, University of St Andrews. The material in Chapter 8 features as part of her thesis. Her work is supervised by Arlene J. Astell. She can be contacted on mellis@computing.dundee.ac.uk.

Paul Hart is Principal Officer (Research) for Sense Scotland. He is also currently enrolled as a PhD student within the School of Psychology at the University of Dundee. The material in Chapter 5 features as part of his thesis. Further details relevant to this chapter can be obtained from him on phart@sensescotland.org.uk.

Jane Horwood is an occupational therapist and independent practitioner of Sensory Integration, based in Peterborough. She can be contacted on childconsultancy@tiscali.co.uk.

Angela Jardine Handley is a Senior Occupational Therapist for Wakefield and Pontefract Learning Disability Psychology Service. She can be contacted on angela.jardine-handley@swyt.nhs.uk.

Martyn C. Jones is a reader based in the School of Nursing and Midwifery at the University of Dundee, and has served as co-supervisor for the PhD thesis described here.

Hilary Kennedy is an Educational Psychologist and Teaching Fellow, based in the School of Education, Social Work and Community Education at the University of Dundee. She is also Director of the Centre for Video Enhanced Reflection on Communication (VEROC) based at the University. She can be contacted on h.a.kennedy@dundee.ac.uk.

Raymond A. R. MacDonald is Professor of Music Psychology in the Department of Psychology at Glasgow Caledonian University. He is also a founder of the George Burt/ Raymond MacDonald Quartet and the Glasgow Improvisers Orchestra. He can be contacted on raymond.macdonald@gcal.ac.uk.

Michelle B. O'Neill was awarded her PhD from the University of Dundee in 2006, funded by the School of Nursing and Midwifery. The material presented in Chapter 4 featured as part of her thesis. Her work was jointly supervised by the co-authors, Martyn C. Jones, a Senior Lecturer based in the School of Nursing and Midwifery, and M. Suzanne Zeedyk, a Senior Lecturer in the School of Psychology. Further details of this work can be obtained from Michelle O'Neill on m.b.oneill@dundee.ac.uk.

Sarah Parry is a 2007 graduate of the University of Manchester, School of Psychology, and Director of the MedLink Romanian Appeal.

Heather Sked received her MSc in Educational Psychology from the University of Dundee in 2006, with material from her research thesis featuring in Chapter 9. She is now employed as an Educational Psychologist by the Highland Council in Scotland. She can be contacted on h.a.sked@dundee.ac.uk.

Colwyn Trevarthen is Professor Emeritus of Child Psychology and Psychobiology, based in the Department of Psychology, in the School of Philosophy, Psychology and Language Sciences, at the University of Edinburgh. He can be contacted on c.trevarthen@ed.ac.uk.

Sarah Walls graduated from the University of Dundee in 2007 with an Honours degree in Psychology, having carried out analyses described in Chapter 6 as part of her final year research dissertations.

M. Suzanne Zeedyk is a Senior Lecturer in Developmental Psychology, in the School of Psychology at the University of Dundee. She can be contacted on m.s.zeedyk@ dundee.ac.uk.

SUBJECT INDEX

AUTHOR INDEX